Care of Cancer Survivors

Editor

KIMBERLY S. PEAIRS

MEDICAL CLINICS
OF NORTH AMERICA

www.medical.theclinics.com

Consulting Editor
BIMAL H. ASHAR

November 2017 • Volume 101 • Number 6

ELSEVIER

1600 John F. Kennedy Boulevard • Suite 1800 • Philadelphia, Pennsylvania, 19103-2899

http://www.theclinics.com

MEDICAL CLINICS OF NORTH AMERICA Volume 101, Number 6
November 2017 ISSN 0025-7125, ISBN-13: 978-0-323-54889-2

Editor: Jessica McCool
Developmental Editor: Alison Swety

Medical Clinics of North America (ISSN 0025-7125) is published bimonthly by Elsevier Inc., 360 Park Avenue South, New York, NY 10010-1710. Months of publication are January, March, May, July, September, and November. Business and editorial offices: 1600 John F. Kennedy Boulevard, Suite 1800, Philadelphia, PA 19103-2899. Periodicals postage paid at New York, NY, and additional mailing offices. Subscription prices are USD $268.00 per year (US individuals), $563.00 per year (US institutions), $100.00 per year (US Students), $330.00 per year (Canadian individuals), $731.00 per year (Canadian institutions), $200.00 per year (Canadian and foreign students), $402.00 per year (foreign individuals), and $731.00 per year (foreign institutions). To receive student/resident rate, orders must be accompanied by name of affiliated institution, date of term, and the signature of program/residency coordinator on institution letterhead. Orders will be billed at individual rate until proof of status is received. Foreign air speed delivery is included in all Clinics' subscription prices. All prices are subject to change without notice. **POSTMASTER:** Send address changes to Medical Clinics of North America, Elsevier Health Sciences Division, Subscription Customer Service, 3251 Riverport Lane, Maryland Heights, MO 63043. **Customer Service: Telephone: 1-800-654-2452** (U.S. and Canada); **1-314-447-8871** (outside U.S. and Canada). **Fax: 314-447-8029. E-mail: journalscustomerserviceusa@elsevier.com** (for print support); **journalsonlinesupport-usa@elsevier.com** (for online support).

Reprints. For copies of 100 or more of articles in this publication, please contact the Commercial Reprints Department, Elsevier Inc., 360 Park Avenue South, New York, NY 10010-1710. Tel.: 212-633-3874; Fax: 212-633-3820; E-mail: reprints@elsevier.com.

Medical Clinics of North America is also published in Spanish by McGraw-Hill Interamericana Editores S. A., P.O. Box 5-237, 06500 Mexico, D.F., Mexico.

Medical Clinics of North America is covered in MEDLINE/PubMed (Index Medicus), Current Contents, ASCA, Excerpta Medica, Science Citation Index, and ISI/BIOMED.

PROGRAM OBJECTIVE
The goal of the *Medical Clinics of North America* is to keep practicing physicians up to date with current clinical practice by providing timely articles reviewing the state of the art in patient care.

TARGET AUDIENCE
All practicing physicians and other healthcare professionals.

LEARNING OBJECTIVES
Upon completion of this activity, participants will be able to:
1. Review issues in hormonal, mental health, and diet issues in cancer care, among others.
2. Discuss fatigue and cognitive issues related to cancer care.
3. Recognize long term and survivorship issues in specific cancer types.

ACCREDITATION
The Elsevier Office of Continuing Medical Education (EOCME) is accredited by the Accreditation Council for Continuing Medical Education (ACCME) to provide continuing medical education for physicians.

The EOCME designates this enduring material for a maximum of 15 *AMA PRA Category 1 Credit*(s)™. Physicians should claim only the credit commensurate with the extent of their participation in the activity.

All other healthcare professionals requesting continuing education credit for this enduring material will be issued a certificate of participation.

DISCLOSURE OF CONFLICTS OF INTEREST
The EOCME assesses conflict of interest with its instructors, faculty, planners, and other individuals who are in a position to control the content of CME activities. All relevant conflicts of interest that are identified are thoroughly vetted by EOCME for fair balance, scientific objectivity, and patient care recommendations. EOCME is committed to providing its learners with CME activities that promote improvements or quality in healthcare and not a specific proprietary business or a commercial interest.

The planning committee, staff, authors and editors listed below have identified no financial relationships or relationships to products or devices they or their spouse/life partner have with commercial interest related to the content of this CME activity:
Nebras Abu Al Hamayel, MBBS, MPH; Bimal H. Ashar, MD, MBA, FACP; Alyssa Berkowitz, MPH; Sharon L. Bober, PhD; Youngjee Choi, MD; Aarati Didwania, MD; Sydney M. Dy, MD, MS; Chidinma C. Ebede, MD; Carmen P. Escalante, MD; Anjali Fortna; Natasha N. Frederick, MD, MPH; Nana Gegechkori, MD, PhD; Mita Sanghavi Goel, MD, MPH; Lindsay Haines, MD; Sarina R. Isenberg, PhD; Yongchang Jang, BS; Kristin Kilbourn, PhD, MPH; Sheetal M. Kircher, MD; Jenny J. Lin, MD, MPH; Arthur Liu, MD, PhD; Leah Logan; Jessica McCool; Karishma Mehra, MD; Kimberly S. Peairs, MD, FACP; Tara Sanft, MD; Jillian L. Simard, MD; Jeyanthi Surendrakumar; Alison Swety; Karen L. Syrjala, PhD; Jean C. Yi, PhD; Eric S. Zhou, PhD.

The planning committee, staff, authors and editors listed below have identified financial relationships or relationships to products or devices they or their spouse/life partner have with commercial interest related to the content of this CME activity:
Linda Overholser, MD, MPH receives royalties/patents from Springer International Publishing, and her spouse/partner has stock ownership in Eli Lilly and Allergan.
Tracy D. Vannorsdall, PhD, ABPP(CN) has research support from Under Armour Women's Health & Breast Cancer Innovation Grant, and receives royalties/patents from PAR, Inc.

UNAPPROVED/OFF-LABEL USE DISCLOSURE
The EOCME requires CME faculty to disclose to the participants:
1. When products or procedures being discussed are off-label, unlabelled, experimental, and/or investigational (not US Food and Drug Administration [FDA] approved); and
2. Any limitations on the information presented, such as data that are preliminary or that represent ongoing research, interim analyses, and/or unsupported opinions. Faculty may discuss information about pharmaceutical agents that is outside of FDA-approved labelling. This information is intended solely for CME and is not intended to promote off-label use of these medications. If you have any questions, contact the medical affairs department of the manufacturer for the most recent prescribing information.

TO ENROLL

To enroll in the *Medical Clinics of North America* Continuing Medical Education program, call customer service at 1-800-654-2452 or sign up online at http://www.theclinics.com/home/cme. The CME program is available to subscribers for an additional annual fee of USD $295.

METHOD OF PARTICIPATION

In order to claim credit, participants must complete the following:

1. Complete enrolment as indicated above.
2. Read the activity.
3. Complete the CME Test and Evaluation. Participants must achieve a score of 70% on the test. All CME Tests and Evaluations must be completed online.

CME INQUIRIES/SPECIAL NEEDS

For all CME inquiries or special needs, please contact elsevierCME@elsevier.com.

MEDICAL CLINICS OF NORTH AMERICA

FORTHCOMING ISSUES

January 2018
Obesity Medicine
Scott Kahan and Robert F. Kushner, *Editors*

March 2018
Urology
Robert E. Brannigan, *Editor*

May 2018
Clinical Examination
Brian T. Garibaldi, *Editor*

RECENT ISSUES

September 2017
Complementary and Integrative Medicine
Robert B. Saper, *Editor*

July 2017
Disease Prevention
Michael P. Pignone and
Kirsten Bibbins-Domingo, *Editors*

May 2017
Emergencies in the Outpatient Setting
Joseph F. Szot, *Editor*

RELATED INTEREST

Primary Care: Clinics in Office Practice, December 2016 (Vol. 43, No. 4)
Hematologic Diseases
Maureen Okam Achebe and Aric Parnes, *Editors*
Available at: http://www.primarycare.theclinics.com/

Contributors

CONSULTING EDITOR

BIMAL H. ASHAR, MD, MBA, FACP
Associate Professor of Medicine, Division of General Internal Medicine, The Johns Hopkins University School of Medicine, Baltimore, Maryland

EDITOR

KIMBERLY S. PEAIRS, MD, FACP
Associate Vice Chair, Ambulatory, Assistant Professor, Department of Medicine, Division of General Internal Medicine, The Johns Hopkins University School of Medicine, Lutherville, Maryland

AUTHORS

NEBRAS ABU AL HAMAYEL, MBBS, MPH
Department of Health Policy and Management, Johns Hopkins Bloomberg School of Public Health, Baltimore, Maryland

ALYSSA BERKOWITZ, MPH
Research Assistant, Department of Medical Oncology, Yale School of Medicine, New Haven, Connecticut

SHARON L. BOBER, PhD
Psychologist, Perini Family Survivors' Center, Director, Sexual Health Program, Dana-Farber Cancer Institute, Assistant Professor, Psychiatry, Harvard Medical School, Boston, Massachusetts

YOUNGJEE CHOI, MD
Assistant Professor, Department of Medicine, Division of General Internal Medicine, The Johns Hopkins University School of Medicine, Baltimore, Maryland

AARATI DIDWANIA, MD
Associate Professor, Department of Medicine, Division of General Internal Medicine and Geriatrics, Northwestern University Feinberg School of Medicine, Chicago, Illinois

SYDNEY M. DY, MD, MS
Primary Care for Cancer Survivors Program, Department of Medicine, The Johns Hopkins University, Baltimore, Maryland

CHIDINMA C. EBEDE, MD
Data Research Coordinator, Department of General Internal Medicine, The University of Texas MD Anderson Cancer Center, Houston, Texas

CARMEN P. ESCALANTE, MD
Professor and Chair, Department of General Internal Medicine, The University of Texas MD Anderson Cancer Center, Houston, Texas

NATASHA N. FREDERICK, MD, MPH
Instructor, Pediatrics, Harvard Medical School, Physician, Pediatric Oncology, Dana-Farber Cancer Institute, Boston, Massachusetts

NANA GEGECHKORI, MD, PhD
Division of General Internal Medicine, Icahn School of Medicine at Mount Sinai, New York, New York

MITA SANGHAVI GOEL, MD, MPH
Assistant Professor, Department of Medicine, Division of General Internal Medicine and Geriatrics, Northwestern University Feinberg School of Medicine, Chicago, Illinois

LINDSAY HAINES, MD
Department of Medicine, Icahn School of Medicine at Mount Sinai, New York, New York

SARINA R. ISENBERG, PhD
Department of Health Behavior and Society, Johns Hopkins Bloomberg School of Public Health, Baltimore, Maryland

YONGCHANG JANG, BS
Research Intern, Department of General Internal Medicine, The University of Texas MD Anderson Cancer Center, Houston, Texas

KRISTIN KILBOURN, PhD, MPH
Associate Professor, Department of Psychology, College of Liberal Arts & Sciences, University of Colorado Denver, Denver, Colorado

SHEETAL M. KIRCHER, MD
Assistant Professor, Department of Medicine, Division of Hematology/Oncology, Northwestern University Feinberg School of Medicine, Chicago, Illinois

JENNY J. LIN, MD, MPH
Associate Professor, Division of General Internal Medicine, Icahn School of Medicine at Mount Sinai, New York, New York

ARTHUR LIU, MD, PhD
Associate Professor, Department of Radiation Oncology, University of Colorado School of Medicine, Aurora, Colorado

KARISHMA MEHRA, MD
Fellow, Department of Medical Oncology, Yale School of Medicine, New Haven, Connecticut

LINDA OVERHOLSER, MD, MPH
Associate Professor, Division of General Internal Medicine, University of Colorado School of Medicine, Aurora, Colorado

TARA SANFT, MD
Assistant Professor of Medicine, Department of Medical Oncology, Yale School of Medicine, New Haven, Connecticut

JILLIAN L. SIMARD, MD
Resident, Internal Medicine, Northwestern Memorial Hospital, Chicago, Illinois

KAREN L. SYRJALA, PhD
Member, Biobehavioral Sciences Department, Fred Hutchinson Cancer Research Center, Department of Psychiatry and Behavioral Sciences, University of Washington School of Medicine, Seattle, Washington

TRACY D. VANNORSDALL, PhD, ABPP(CN)
Assistant Professor, Departments of Psychiatry and Behavioral Sciences, and Neurology, The Johns Hopkins University School of Medicine, Baltimore, Maryland

JEAN C. YI, PhD
Senior Staff Scientist, Biobehavioral Sciences, Fred Hutchinson Cancer Research Center, Seattle, Washington

ERIC S. ZHOU, PhD
Psychologist, Perini Family Survivors' Center, Dana-Farber Cancer Institute, Instructor, Pediatrics, Harvard Medical School, Boston, Massachusetts

Contents

Foreword: A Lifelong Battle   xv

Bimal H. Ashar

Preface: The Many Facets of Cancer Survivorship   xvii

Kimberly S. Peairs

Care Coordination and Transitions of Care   1041

Youngjee Choi

> Care coordination and effective transitions of care are essential for high-quality care in cancer survivors. Aspects of care that require coordination include cancer surveillance, managing the effects of cancer and its treatment, and preventive care, including screening for new cancers, with the clinician responsible for each aspect of care clearly defined. There are many barriers to transitioning and coordinating care across cancer specialists and primary care physicians; possible solutions include survivorship care plans and certain care models. Improving these areas, along with survivorship care training and education, may lead to more effective care coordination and transitions in the future.

Long-Term and Latent Side Effects of Specific Cancer Types   1053

Nana Gegechkori, Lindsay Haines, and Jenny J. Lin

> Although many cancer survivors diagnosed with early-stage disease will outlive their cancer, they may continue to experience long-term and/or latent side effects due to cancer treatment. Many of these side effects are common and contribute to worse quality of life, morbidity, and mortality for cancer survivors. This article summarizes the treatment side effects for several of the most prevalent cancers in the United States.

Survivorship Issues in Adolescent and Young Adult Oncology   1075

Linda Overholser, Kristin Kilbourn, and Arthur Liu

> Adolescent and young adult (AYA) individuals with a history of cancer make up a fraction of the total number of cancer survivors in the United States, but they represent a population with needs distinct from either the childhood or the older adult cancer populations. Fertility concerns, psychosocial factors, and health care access are just a few of the distinguishing characteristics. Caring for AYA cancer survivors presents unique opportunities for primary care providers to collaborate with oncology colleagues to minimize the long-term cancer burden.

Cancer-Related Fatigue in Cancer Survivorship   1085

Chidinma C. Ebede, Yongchang Jang, and Carmen P. Escalante

> Cancer-related fatigue (CRF) significantly interferes with usual functioning because of the distressing sense of physical, emotional, and cognitive exhaustion. Assessment of CRF is important and should be performed during the initial cancer diagnosis, throughout cancer treatment, and after treatment using a fatigue scoring scale (mild-severe). The general approach to CRF management applies to cancer survivors at all fatigue levels and includes education, counseling, and other strategies. Nonpharmacologic interventions include psychosocial interventions, exercise, yoga, physically based therapy, dietary management, and sleep therapy. Pharmacologic interventions include psychostimulants. Antidepressants may also benefit when CRF is accompanied by depression.

Anxiety and Depression in Cancer Survivors   1099

Jean C. Yi and Karen L. Syrjala

> Most cancer survivors adjust well to life after cancer, but some experience persisting negative mood, such as cancer-related fears, posttraumatic stress, anxiety, or depression. Mood fluctuations may not reach criteria for a clinical diagnosis, but subclinical symptoms can interfere with quality of life. Women, adolescents, and young adults are particularly at risk for mood disturbances. Behavioral interventions, such as cognitive behavioral therapy and pharmacologic treatments, can effectively treat these distressing emotions. Much of the research on managing emotional needs after cancer has been completed with breast cancer survivors, and more work is needed with diverse groups of survivors.

Cognitive Changes Related to Cancer Therapy   1115

Tracy D. Vannorsdall

> A growing population of cancer survivors is at risk for acute and long-term consequences resulting from cancer and its treatment. Cancer-related cognitive impairment (CRCI) typically manifests as modest deficits in attention, processing speed, executive functioning, and memory, which may persist for decades after treatment. Although some risk factors for CRCI are largely immutable (eg, genetics and demographic factors), there are many other contributors to CRCI that when appropriately addressed can result in improved cognitive functioning and quality of life. Neuropsychological assessment can help identify patient cognitive strengths and weaknesses, target psychological and behavioral contributors to CRCI, and guide treatment interventions.

Hormonal Changes and Sexual Dysfunction   1135

Eric S. Zhou, Natasha N. Frederick, and Sharon L. Bober

> Sexual dysfunction is a common concern for many patients with cancer after treatment. Hormonal changes as a result of cancer-directed therapy can affect both male and female sexual health. This has the potential to significantly affect patients' quality of life but is underreported and undertreated in the oncology setting. This article discusses commonly reported sexual issues and the role that hormonal changes play in this dysfunction.

Although medical and psychosocial intervention strategies exist, there is a clear need for further research to formally develop programming that can assist people whose sexual health has been affected by cancer treatment.

Diet, Physical Activity, and Body Weight in Cancer Survivorship   1151

Karishma Mehra, Alyssa Berkowitz, and Tara Sanft

Diet, physical activity, and body weight have been shown to play an important role in cancer survivorship. The impact of each of these lifestyle factors differs slightly among cancer types, and adherence to recommended diet and physical activity guidelines has been associated with positive outcomes, including decrease in the risk of cancer recurrence and improvement of quality of life. Although there are compelling data that appropriate diet, physical activity, and body weight have beneficial effects in cancer survivorship, additional trials are needed to understand the relationship.

Screening for Recurrence and Secondary Cancers   1167

Jillian L. Simard, Sheetal M. Kircher, Aarati Didwania, and Mita Sanghavi Goel

The population of adult cancer survivors is increasing over time and they are at risk of developing recurrent and secondary cancers, even years after completion of treatment. Posttreatment care of survivors is increasingly the responsibility of primary care providers. Surveillance for recurrence and screening for secondary malignancies related to treatment depend largely on the primary malignancy, treatment regimen, and presence of a hereditary cancer syndrome, such as a BRCA mutation. This article presents surveillance strategies for the most common malignancies.

Palliative Care for Cancer Survivors   1181

Sydney M. Dy, Sarina R. Isenberg, and Nebras Abu Al Hamayel

The palliative care approach for survivors begins with comprehensive assessment of communication and advance care planning needs and the physical, psychological and psychiatric, social, spiritual and religious, and cultural domains. Communication and decision making about difficult issues should include responding to emotions, planning for future communication needs, and considering reasons for miscommunication. Key palliative approaches to symptom management include addressing physical and psychosocial concerns, and using nonpharmacologic approaches first or together with medications. Physicians should address advance care planning in older cancer survivors and those at significant risk of recurrence and mortality, ideally through ongoing conversations in a longitudinal care relationship.

Foreword

A Lifelong Battle

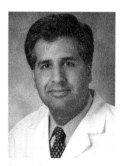

Bimal H. Ashar, MD, MBA, FACP
Consulting Editor

For many years, the term "cancer survivor" referred to a patient who had been diagnosed with cancer, treated, and remained cancer free for at least 5 years. This clinical definition rather arbitrarily categorized patients with cancer as either "victims" or "survivors." In 1986, the National Coalition for Cancer Survivorship (NCCS) redefined this term to encompass all patients with cancer, from the time of diagnosis through the end of their lives. This expanded view was designed to change the way that people with cancer talked about their diagnosis and to empower them to be active participants in their care. The NCCS later expanded the definition to recognize the impact of cancer on survivors' family members, friends, and caregivers.

As of January 2016, there were approximately 15.5 million cancer survivors in the United States, representing nearly 5% of the population. Partially due to advances in detection and treatment as well as an aging population, the number of cancer survivors is expected to grow to over 20 million by 2026. Despite the large numbers of individuals afflicted by cancer, data show that these patients often receive suboptimal care, perhaps due to gaps in knowledge or ill-defined roles and insufficient communication between oncologists and primary care physicians. In addition to receiving routine preventive care, cancer survivors who are no longer in treatment face unique health risks that require them to be monitored for recurrence of their primary tumor, screened for secondary cancers, and evaluated for late physical and psychological effects of their cancer and its treatment.

In this issue of *Medical Clinics of North America*, Dr Kimberly Peairs has assembled an accomplished group of experts in the field of cancer survivorship to address some

Med Clin N Am 101 (2017) xv–xvi
http://dx.doi.org/10.1016/j.mcna.2017.08.002
0025-7125/17/© 2017 Published by Elsevier Inc.

medical.theclinics.com

of the potential gaps in physicians' knowledge. It is hoped that enhancing the provider's armamentarium will lead to gains on the battlefield.

Bimal H. Ashar, MD, MBA, FACP
Division of General Internal Medicine
Johns Hopkins University School of Medicine
601 North Caroline Street
#7143
Baltimore, MD 21287, USA

E-mail address:
Bashar1@jhmi.edu

Preface

The Many Facets of Cancer Survivorship

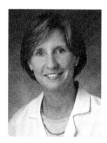

Kimberly S. Peairs, MD, FACP
Editor

With improvements in cancer screening and treatment, a diagnosis of cancer for many patients is one of chronic disease or a cure with long-term sequelae. There are now presently over 15 million cancer survivors living in the United States, and numbers are expected to grow.[1] In 2006, an Institute of Medicine report defined cancer survivorship as a distinct phase of care with essential components of the care.[2] That report outlined some of the challenges these patients may face as well as the gaps in care delivery. In this issue of the *Medical Clinics of North America*, many of the issues that are unique to cancer survivors are reviewed with a fresh look at the most current literature on the subject.

The spectrum of cancer survivorship care is encompassed by transitions of care and care coordination that can be complex. Good communication between primary care providers and oncology practitioners is paramount. The challenges presented by our health system and models of care delivery are explored.

The potential long-term and latent side effects of the most common treatments are outlined. In particular, reviews on anxiety and depression, cognitive changes, sexual dysfunction, and fatigue related to cancer and its treatment are presented. The interplay of diet, physical activity, and weight is relevant for not only prevention of cancer but also cancer-related outcomes. An overview of the evidence-based literature as it pertains to some of the more common cancer types is included.

The unique needs of adolescent and young adult cancer survivors are reviewed. These individuals will likely be followed in adult care settings, increasing the importance of educating our primary care providers about this topic. Appropriate surveillance for cancer recurrence and screening for secondary cancers creates great stress for patients, and the most up-to-date guidelines for the most common tumor types are covered. Finally, the importance of addressing palliative care issues during the cancer continuum is discussed.

Med Clin N Am 101 (2017) xvii–xviii
http://dx.doi.org/10.1016/j.mcna.2017.08.001
0025-7125/17/© 2017 Published by Elsevier Inc.

medical.theclinics.com

I am appreciative of the work the authors have put forward to present this issue on cancer survivorship and am hopeful these reviews will assist with improvements in the care delivery.

Kimberly S. Peairs, MD, FACP
Associate Vice Chair, Ambulatory
Assistant Professor
Department of Medicine
Division of General Internal Medicine
The Johns Hopkins University School of Medicine
Suite 325, 10753 Falls Road
Lutherville, MD 20193, USA

E-mail address:
kpeairs@jhmi.edu

REFERENCES

1. Miller KD, Siegel RL, Lin CC, et al. Cancer treatment and survivorship statistics, 2016. CA Cancer J Clin 2016;66(5):271–89.
2. Hewitt M, Greenfield S, Stovall E. From cancer patient to cancer survivor: lost in translation. Washington, DC: National Academies Press; 2006.

Care Coordination and Transitions of Care

Youngjee Choi, MD*

KEYWORDS

- Coordination of care • Transitions of care • Cancer survivorship

KEY POINTS

- Care coordination and transitions of care between cancer specialists and primary care physicians (PCPs) are variable.
- Barriers include lack of explicit clinician responsibility for care components, different preferences for care models, and oncologists' perception of PCP competence to care for cancer survivors.
- A survivorship care plan may help communication between cancer specialists and PCPs, and thus, care coordination and transitions.
- A model of shared care between cancer specialists and PCPs seems to improve survivors' receipt of cancer-related and preventive care.
- Improvements in survivorship care education may facilitate improved care coordination and transitions.

INTRODUCTION

Care coordination and effective transitions of care are essential for providing high-quality care in many chronic diseases, only recently have they been given significant attention in cancer survivorship. In 2006, the Institute of Medicine (IOM) report, "From Cancer Care to Cancer Survivor: Lost in Transition," described the fragmentation of care experienced by cancer survivors and put forth as 1 of 4 essential components of survivorship care, the care coordination between cancer specialists and primary care physicians (PCP).[1] This fundamental aspect of care becomes even more critical in light of anticipated oncologist and PCP shortages, the physicians primarily responsible for cancer survivorship care.[2–4] Effective models of care and efficient processes of coordinating care for cancer survivors will become ever more important.

Conflicts of Interest: None. This author receives no funding from public, commercial, or not-for-profit sectors.
Department of Medicine, Division of General Internal Medicine, The Johns Hopkins University School of Medicine, Baltimore, MD, USA
* 10753 Falls Road, Suite 325, Lutherville, MD 21093.
E-mail address: ychoi47@jhmi.edu

Med Clin N Am 101 (2017) 1041–1051
http://dx.doi.org/10.1016/j.mcna.2017.06.001
0025-7125/17/© 2017 Elsevier Inc. All rights reserved.

In the following article, the following are reviewed:

1. Components of care coordination and transitions
2. The current gaps in care coordination and transitions
3. Barriers and facilitators of care coordination and transitions including survivorship care plans (SCPs) and models of care
4. Future considerations to improve care coordination and transitions.

CARE COORDINATION AND TRANSITIONS OF CARE: WHO, WHAT, AND DESIGNATING RESPONSIBILITY

Care coordination has been defined as "the deliberate organization of patient care activities between two or more participants... involved in a patient's care to facilitate the appropriate delivery of health care services... often managed by the exchange of information among participants responsible for different aspects of care."[5] To maximize coordination based on this definition, it is important to identify the main clinicians involved, specify the care components, and delineate responsibility.

The clinicians involved include the various cancer specialists (medical oncologists, radiation oncologists, surgeons) and PCPs, with much of the literature focusing on the role of medical oncologists and PCPs. As highlighted in a study by Haggstrom and colleagues,[6] cancer survivors are often seeing multiple clinicians for their care. After 2 to 5 years from their initial diagnosis, 40% of surveyed colorectal cancer survivors were seeing at least 2 clinicians (most often a medical oncologist as their main physician), and nearly 20% were seeing at least 4 clinicians, including non–cancer physicians such as gastroenterologists.

Essential components of care have been delineated in the 2006 IOM report as the following: *prevention* of recurrent cancers, new cancers, and late effects; *surveillance* of recurrent cancers and late effects; and *intervention* for the effects of cancer and its treatment.[1] Many studies have included preventive care efforts such as vaccinations and other health maintenance measures as relevant components of survivorship care.[7–9] However, physicians are not routinely addressing survivorship care with patients with cancer. In the Survey of Physicians' Attitudes Regarding the Care of Cancer Survivors (SPARCCS), a survey of more than 2000 oncologists and PCPs, approximately two-thirds of oncologists, and one-fifth of PCPs regularly discussed survivorship care recommendations with their patients.[10]

Clinician responsibility, or designating specific aspects of care to particular clinicians, helps ensure that care is actually delivered. For example, in the SPARCCS data, the oncologists who preferred shared care with other clinicians were less likely to discuss survivorship care and clinician responsibility with patients,[10] suggesting that a diffusion of responsibility without clearly delineated roles can lead to further poor coordination of care. Despite the importance of delineating clinician responsibility, this aspect of care coordination is infrequently addressed. Snyder and colleagues[11] have suggested that less cancer screening may be occurring as survivors see their oncologist less frequently over time because responsibility for preventive care has not been explicitly transitioned to the PCP.

GAPS IN CARE COORDINATION AND TRANSITIONS OF CARE
Primary Care Physician Perspective

Soon after the IOM report, Nissen and colleagues[12] reported on gaps in care coordination perceived by PCPs for breast and colorectal cancer survivors. More than 50% of PCPs surveyed rated the transition of care from oncologists as poor or fair. In addition, 57% to 74% of PCPs were unsure how to provide follow-up surveillance, and more than 40% of PCPs were concerned about missed or duplicated care with the oncologist and were unclear regarding who was responsible for preventive health care. PCPs also expressed concern over lack of patient education about appropriate future clinical triage (21% stated patients contacted the oncologist for problems better addressed by the PCP, whereas 40% stated the patients contacted the PCP for problems better addressed by the oncologist). PCPs suggested that more communication from oncologists, particularly in their recommendations for surveillance testing, would improve care transitions. Other studies have confirmed that PCPs are willing to provide follow-up surveillance care if guidelines are provided.[13–15] In a survey of Canadian PCPs regarding their survivors of prostate cancer, breast cancer, colorectal cancer, and lymphoma, PCPs reported willingness to assume complete responsibility for survivorship care, on average 2 to 3 years after treatment completion.[16]

In a recent systematic review of the relationship between medical oncologists and PCPs, one of the themes seen in the literature was poor or delayed communication with the PCP.[13] Up to 60% of PCPs in studies reported communication was inadequate in content and too infrequent. Oncologists suggested they could communicate better, but only 40% of oncologists reported providing regular communication to PCPs. Specifically, a formal hand-off of survivorship care to the PCP appeared to be lacking, with only 56% of PCPs in one study reporting explicit communication from the oncologist, whereas in another study, more than half of PCPs reported this communication was infrequent.[13] Besides new requirements to provide SCPs as discussed later, there are no other standards for how oncologists and PCPs should communicate on an ongoing basis. In terms of modes of communication, PCPs have expressed that they prefer phone calls or e-mail.[13,17]

Cancer Specialist Perspective

In the systematic review previously described, another identified theme was the preference of cancer specialists to have an oncology-centric model of care, including domains typically considered primary care.[13] Some oncologists considered their patients too ill to go to multiple physicians, whereas other oncologists felt uncertain of PCPs' knowledge and skill to provide effective survivorship care. Oncologists have also expressed uncertainty in who is managing preventive care (42%) and concerns of duplicated care (56%), more frequently than PCPs.[18] In another qualitative study, medical oncologists specifically wanted better comorbidity management from their PCP colleagues[19] (cancer survivors have less than recommended follow-up visits for diabetes, cardiac problems, and respiratory comorbidities compared with matched controls without cancer).[20] However, this role was unclear to PCPs, who felt their care took a back seat during active cancer treatment.[19] There was no literature addressing communication from PCPs to oncologists.[13]

Patient Perspective

In a study of colorectal cancer survivors, patients who saw their oncologist as their main physician were more likely to report seeing a doctor for follow-up tests, whereas those most often seeing their PCP were more likely to report follow-up for lifestyle and diet.[6] Despite perceiving that these areas of care were addressed, when asked explicitly about the physician responsible for different aspects of their care, patients have been less certain. Interviewed breast and colorectal cancer survivors expressed confusion with clinician roles and responsibilities for their general care as well as cancer-related care. Patients reporting good continuity of care felt they had a designated point of contact (whether a navigator, oncology nurse, or

PCP) and had received care in programs where multiple clinicians could easily be accessed together, as in a comprehensive care program.[21] In another study, patients with multiple medical comorbidities, with lower health literacy, or who lacked a PCP or designated cancer care coordinator perceived poorer care coordination.[22] Despite efforts to improve care coordination including with SCPs, survivors have reported that psychosocial concerns and long-term effects are still inadequately addressed.[23]

BARRIERS AND FACILITATORS OF CARE COORDINATION AND TRANSITIONS OF CARE
Barriers

There are several differences between oncologists and PCPs that may be barriers to effective care coordination and willingness to transition care to the PCP: (1) perceived roles in survivorship care, (2) preferred models of care, and (3) differences in perceived skills and knowledge of survivorship care.

Oncologists and PCPs have significantly differing viewpoints of their respective roles in survivorship care. In one study looking at which physician (oncologist or PCP) should have main responsibility for primary cancer surveillance, new cancer screening, and general preventive care, oncologists and PCPs had 3%, 44%, and 51% concordance, respectively, in their assignment of physician responsibility; in general, both oncologists and PCPs claimed more responsibility for each aspect of care.[24] Nearly 70% of oncologists in SPARCCS thought they predominately provide follow-up care for their cancer survivors, whereas PCPs stated predominately providing or comanaging care 40% of the time; these reports suggest the possibility of duplicated care by these 2 physician groups, who both assume responsibility and may be unaware of what other physicians are providing.[25] Similarly, in SPARCCS, nearly 60% of oncologists preferred a cancer specialist–led model, whereas PCPs predominately favored a shared care model (40%).[26]

Oncologists also have less confidence in PCPs' ability to provide cancer survivorship care. Whereas 58% to 75% of PCPs felt that PCPs in general had the skills to address the effects of cancer and cancer treatment or provide surveillance and evaluation for breast and colorectal cancer recurrence, only 23% to 38% of oncologists agreed. It should be noted, however, that when PCPs were asked about their personal confidence in these domains, only 23% of PCPs expressed high confidence in addressing late effects of cancer, and 40% were very confident in knowing the tests to work-up cancer recurrence (interestingly, both oncologists and PCPs recommended more surveillance testing than guidelines suggest, reflecting knowledge gaps across clinicians).

Oncologists' less favorable perceptions of PCPs' abilities are despite data suggesting equivalent outcomes in cancer survivors who are followed exclusively by PCPs versus oncologists, and perhaps even improved receipt of cancer-related and preventive care with PCP comanagement. In a randomized, controlled trial of patients with early-stage breast cancer who completed active treatment, there were no differences in clinical endpoints (death or recurrence) or quality-of-life outcomes in those followed by their cancer center or PCP exclusively.[27]

Although there has been limited evidence to support shared care for chronic diseases in prior Cochrane Reviews,[28] more recent studies suggest cancer survivors may benefit from both oncologist and PCP involvement. Studies have shown that individuals seeing both their oncologist and their PCP received more cancer-related and preventive care compared with individuals seeing only either clinician. Specifically, in colorectal cancer survivors, preventive care, including influenza vaccination, cholesterol screening, bone density, and screening for new cancers, were more likely to occur in patients who saw both their oncologist and their PCP.[7,11,20] Surveillance colonoscopy was more likely to occur in colorectal cancer survivors who saw their PCP.[29] Similar patterns in preventive care as well as surveillance mammography were seen for patients with breast cancer who saw their oncologist and PCP, compared with only a single physician.[8,30,31] Cancer survivors with other medical comorbidities were also less likely to have their comorbid conditions managed appropriately without PCP visits.[20,32]

Despite data showing the value of PCP care in cancer survivors, oncologist and PCP viewpoints differed regarding their roles and models of care. Especially by feeling uncertain of PCPs' knowledge or skill, oncologists may be hesitant to comanage patients or transition patients to exclusive care by their PCP. Notably, oncologists who had more positive views of PCPs' ability to provide survivorship care were more likely to comanage with PCPs.[25]

Facilitators

Medical oncologists and PCPs have reported that the electronic medical record (EMR) facilitates communication within an integrated system, although it remains difficult to communicate effectively with outside clinicians.[19]

Explicit conversations regarding clinician responsibility additionally seem to aid in care receipt. When patients reported they had discussed clinician responsibility for cancer follow-up or general medical care with their oncologists, patient and oncologist expectations were better aligned, and this was correlated with more frequent receipt of influenza vaccinations and routine physicals.[33] These conversations suggests that improved communication between patients and oncologists, by better synchronizing expectations, can improve care coordination and receipt.

The Survivorship Care Plan

One solution proposed to bridge some of the gaps in coordination and transitions of care is the SCP. The use of an SCP as a communication tool was one of the 10 recommendations proposed by the IOM to facilitate survivorship care. SCPs may include 2 components: (1) a treatment summary, and (2) a follow-up plan of care that outlines surveillance testing (type, frequency, and duration), preventive care recommendations, and potential psychosocial and financial concerns.

Although the intent is appropriate, the acceptance of SCPs has not been straightforward because there has been debate over the purpose and format of the SCP. Is it primarily to provide important information to the patient, or to be a communication tool for clinicians, perhaps in lieu of a traditional letter from a consultant? What constitutes an effective SCP without it being overly burdensome? Some have also proposed that the SCP should differ based on the anticipated model of care (shared care vs complete transition to the PCP).[34] In general, cancer survivors, oncologists, and PCPs prefer the SCP to be timed within the first 6 months after treatment completion.[23]

The American Society for Clinical Oncology (ASCO) organized a consensus conference with multidisciplinary stakeholders to discuss and improve the SCP. They focused on the key components for both the treatment summary and the follow-up care plan from the more extensive list initially proposed by the IOM report.[1,35] The revised ASCO SCP templates produced were simplified versions with more practical application. Other organizations have constructed SCP templates, such as Journey Forward and the Livestrong care plan.[23]

Implementation of Survivorship Care Plans

Despite the potential benefits of using SCPs, they are inconsistently completed in practice. A study of Livestrong Survivorship centers, which included both comprehensive cancer centers and community-based centers, showed that their SCPs contained only about 60% of IOM-recommended components. Although their SCP template included assignment of clinician responsibility for surveillance and screening tests, clinician responsibility was addressed in SCPs 17% to 54% of the time. Furthermore, 30% of Livestrong sites did not routinely share SCPs with PCPs.[36] In a randomized, controlled study attempting to provide PCPs with SCPs versus usual care, only a third of PCPs in the intervention arm reported receiving an SCP.[37] In another study of the National Cancer Institute (NCI)-designated cancer centers, only 43% of sites provided an SCP to their breast and colorectal cancer survivors.[38] In SPARCCS, which was mostly community physicians, fewer than 10% of oncologists reported providing a written SCP to survivors,[10] whereas 24% and 45% did not provide a treatment summary or follow-up care plan, respectively, to PCPs; 27% of oncologists did not delineate physician responsibility with the other physicians involved.[25]

The ASCO consensus work group reiterated several barriers to SCP implementation reported in the literature: the length of time required to prepare the SCP, lack of reimbursement for this time, and limited "partnership between oncology and PCPs to facilitate communication and coordination of care." A component of the "partnership" hurdle was that some patients did not have a prior PCP, and it was suggested that cancer centers have an established referral base of PCPs for these situations.[35] Other reported barriers in the literature include sustainability and lack of a standardized SCP format.[23] Shorter, standardized templates integrated into the EMR may help completions rates by cancer care teams.

Since 2015, the American College of Surgeon's Commission on Cancer, an accreditation board for cancer programs in the United States, has been taking steps to implement survivorship care standards based on the IOM report. Specifically, they have set requirements for institutions to provide SCPs to a percentage of eligible patients, reaching at least 75% by 2019,[39] despite the lack of definitive evidence that SCPs improve care coordination and transitions for cancer survivors.

Effectiveness of Survivorship Care Plans

SCPs appear to improve perceived care coordination by both patients and clinicians. In a study by Palmer and colleagues,[40] breast cancer survivors felt care coordination was significantly better after receiving an SCP as well as physician knowledge and knowledge for self-management, and 90% reported general satisfaction with their SCP. A review of studies on SCPs from 2006 to 2013 suggested that SCPs lead to PCPs perceiving better care coordination and communication as well.[41] Notably in SPARCCS, although only 21% of PCPs reported discussing survivorship care with their patients, PCPs who received an SCP were more than 9 times as likely to do so.[10] PCPs who received a treatment summary or follow-up care plan were less likely to report inadequate knowledge or training to manage cancer survivors.[18]

However, there is limited evidence that SCPs directly improve coordination or transitions of care, with few studies adequately designed or powered to assess their effectiveness.[42] A *Cochrane Review* in 2012 showed that there was no clear intervention demonstrating improvements in care coordination.[43] There have been several negative randomized controlled trials looking at the efficacy of SCPs in care coordination and patient-reported outcomes.[44,45] Future studies may be able to overcome these limitations of study design, by refocusing the question of what SCPs can achieve as a communication tool among clinicians. As one editorial stated, "care plans are vehicles for communication and coordination of care, nothing more" and do not substitute for good care.[42] Stricker and colleagues[36] concluded that SCPs are not likely to overcome fragmented survivorship care, but need to be part of a larger comprehensive plan.

MODELS OF CARE

Fig. 1 from Dossett and colleagues[13] illustrates the relationship and components involved in care coordination between the PCP and cancer specialist. As part of this dynamic, various models of care have been proposed for cancer survivors. A recent systematic review outlined formal survivorship models centered in oncology that were described in the literature. Models appear to be divided by several categories, including cancer type, setting (within or separate from cancer centers), clinician type (physician, advanced practitioner, registered nurse), consultative (one-time) versus longitudinal services, and in some cases, a specific purpose (eg, transition clinic to bridge patients to the PCP). The most resource-intensive model is based on multidisciplinary clinics for childhood cancer survivors and has been suggested for small groups of patients with very complex needs.[47] Although risk-based follow-up has been suggested in guidelines for childhood cancer survivors,[48] a patient's risk of recurrence and late effects has not been explicitly considered in models of care for adult cancer survivorship.[46,47] One of the conclusions of the systematic review was that models are very individualized to each institution and that common-alities may be difficult to find and assess.[46]

More recently, models of care have been proposed centering around the PCP, with PCPs working in 2 different roles.[49] These roles include PCPs acting as "oncogener-alists" who help transition patients from cancer specialists to a community PCP, and as comanagers in shared care, where an on-going collaboration is maintained between oncology specialists and PCPs. The latter may be more viable for the vast majority of patients (85%) who are treated outside of an NCI-designated cancer

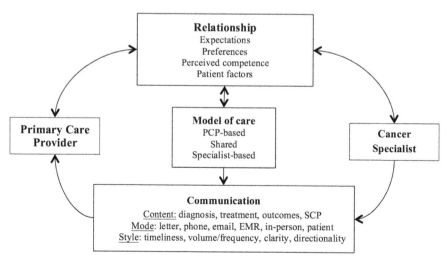

Fig. 1. Model of the PCP–cancer specialist relationship. (*From* Dossett LA, Hudson JN, Morris AM, et al. The primary care provider (PCP)-cancer specialist relationship: a systematic review and mixed-methods meta-synthesis. CA Cancer J Clin 2016;67(2):8; with permission.)

center.[50] In situations where patients are being transitioned to the PCP, coordination of care means having the cancer specialists communicate a surveillance plan and management of the current and anticipated effects of cancer and its treatment (ie, an SCP), in addition to a pathway to refer back to quickly if recurrence is suspected. In situations of shared care, the most important aspect of care coordination may be having roles clearly delineated for the cancer specialists and PCPs, with frequent communication among clinicians to avoid duplication and gaps in care.

Characterization and evaluation of different models have been limited in the literature and even more sparse in regards to care coordination.[46] Care coordination among clinicians was not directly examined in any studies of models of care, and transitions were studied in the context of SCPs in only 3 trials.

Patients seem to prefer either a shared care model or a cancer-specialist model, with only 8% preferring their PCP to be the sole clinician for their cancer care in one study (although this was not controlled for stage of disease).[22] In a survey of nearly 1000 cancer survivors within their first 2 years of diagnosis, 91% of patients expressed the expectation that their oncologist would have a substantial role in their cancer surveillance, compared with 33% for their PCPs to have a similar role.[24] In a study of young adult cancer survivors in the United Kingdom, survivors preferred follow-up care with a cancer specialist above their PCP.[51] Patient preference for continued oncology care was also suggested in a randomized, controlled trial of survivorship care where one arm was followed up solely by their PCP; 45% of potential patients declined study participation.[27]

In the limited number of studies regarding models transitioning from an oncologist to care solely by a PCP, there were no significant differences in clinical event rates related to recurrence, time to recurrence, adherence to guidelines, and patient-reported outcomes.[47] Given this evidence, and the benefits of overall care receipt (including cancer surveillance) with shared care or PCP involvement as discussed above, encouraging medical oncologists to help patients feel more comfortable and confident with PCP management may be an important factor in transitioning patients effectively from oncology.

FUTURE CONSIDERATIONS

Increasing training and education in survivorship care can be one strategy to improve care coordination. In SPARCCS, oncologists who had received training on survivorship care were more likely to discuss survivorship and clinician responsibility. Of the PCPs who had attended a course on the care of childhood cancer survivors, 97% were very willing to share care in these patients, and 64% even felt primarily responsible for their survivorship care.[52] In a large study of mostly community PCPs, more than 50% did not feel there were guidelines for PCPs on survivorship management, and nearly half felt they had inadequate training.[15] Having practical resources easily accessible for busy clinicians will be necessary to bridge this educational gap. One such example is "Follow-up after treatment for breast cancer: practical guide to survivorship care for family physicians" recently published in the *Canadian Family Physician*.[53] As noted by Dossett and colleagues,[13] primary care training programs should include education in caring for cancer survivors, and continuing medical education courses should be provided for practicing PCPs.

SUMMARY

Care coordination and transitions of care between cancer specialists and PCPs need continual improvement. Aspects of care that require coordination include cancer surveillance, management of the effects of cancer and its treatment, and preventive care, including screening for new cancers. Barriers to care coordination include lack of explicit clinician responsibility for care components, different preferences for care models, and oncologists' perception of PCP competence to care for survivors. An SCP may help communication between cancer specialists and PCPs, and a model of shared care between cancer specialists and PCPs seems to improve survivors' receipt of cancer-related and preventive care. Improvements in survivorship care education may lead to more effective care coordination and transitions in the future.

REFERENCES

1. Hewitt M, Greenfield S, Stovall E. From cancer patient to cancer survivor: lost in translation. Washington, DC: National Academies Press; 2006.
2. Erikson C, Salsberg E, Forte G, et al. Future supply and demand for oncologists: challenges to assuring access to oncology services. J Oncol Pract 2007;3(2): 79–86.
3. Yang W, Williams JH, Hogan PF, et al. Projected supply of and demand for oncologists and radiation oncologists through 2025: an aging, better-insured population will result in shortage. J Oncol Pract 2014;10(1):39–45.
4. Petterson SM, Liaw WR, Tran C, et al. Estimating the residency expansion required to avoid projected primary care physician shortages by 2035. Ann Fam Med 2015;13(2):107–14.
5. McDonald KM, Sundaram V, Bravata DM, et al, editors. Closing the quality gap: a critical analysis of quality improvement strategies. Volume 7—care coordination. Rockville (MD): Agency for Healthcare Research and Quality; 2007.
6. Haggstrom DA, Arora NK, Helft P, et al. Follow-up care delivery among colorectal cancer survivors most often seen by primary and subspecialty care physicians. J Gen Intern Med 2009;24(Suppl 2):S472–9.
7. Snyder CF, Earle CC, Herbert RJ, et al. Trends in follow-up and preventive care for colorectal cancer survivors. J Gen Intern Med 2008;23(3):254–9.
8. Snyder CF, Frick KD, Kantsiper ME, et al. Prevention, screening, and surveillance care for breast cancer survivors compared with controls: changes from 1998 to 2002. J Clin Oncol 2009;27(7):1054–61.
9. Snyder CF, Frick KD, Herbert RJ, et al. Preventive care in prostate cancer patients: following diagnosis and for five-year survivors. J Cancer Surviv 2011; 5(3):283–91.
10. Blanch-Hartigan D, Forsythe LP, Alfano CM, et al. Provision and discussion of survivorship care plans among cancer survivors: results of a nationally representative survey of oncologists and primary care physicians. J Clin Oncol 2014; 32(15):1578–85.
11. Snyder CF, Earle CC, Herbert RJ, et al. Preventive care for colorectal cancer survivors: a 5-year longitudinal study. J Clin Oncol 2008;26(7):1073–9.
12. Nissen MJ, Beran MS, Lee MW, et al. Views of primary care providers on follow-up care of cancer patients. Fam Med 2007;39(7):477–82.
13. Dossett LA, Hudson JN, Morris AM, et al. The primary care provider (PCP)-cancer specialist relationship: a systematic review and mixed-methods meta-synthesis. CA Cancer J Clin 2016;67(2):156–69.
14. Papagrigoriadis S, Koreli A. The needs of general practitioners in the follow-up of patients with colorectal cancer. Eur J Surg Oncol 2001;27(6):541–4.
15. Bober SL, Recklitis CJ, Campbell EG, et al. Caring for cancer survivors: a survey of primary care physicians. Cancer 2009;115(18 Suppl):4409–18.

16. Del Giudice ME, Grunfeld E, Harvey BJ, et al. Primary care physicians' views of routine follow-up care of cancer survivors. J Clin Oncol 2009;27(20):3338–45.

17. Shen MJ, Binz-Scharf M, D'Agostino T, et al. A mixed-methods examination of communication between oncologists and primary care providers among primary care physicians in underserved communities. Cancer 2015;121(6):908–15.

18. Virgo KS, Lerro CC, Klabunde CN, et al. Barriers to breast and colorectal cancer survivorship care: perceptions of primary care physicians and medical oncologists in the United States. J Clin Oncol 2013;31(18):2322–36.

19. Sada YH, Street RL Jr, Singh H, et al. Primary care and communication in shared cancer care: a qualitative study. Am J Manag Care 2011;17(4):259–65.

20. Earle CC, Neville BA. Under use of necessary care among cancer survivors. Cancer 2004;101(8):1712–9.

21. Easley J, Miedema B, Carroll JC, et al. Patients' experiences with continuity of cancer care in Canada: results from the CanIMPACT study. Can Fam Physician 2016;62(10):821–7.

22. Durcinoska I, Young JM, Solomon MJ. Patterns and predictors of colorectal cancer care coordination: a population-based survey of Australian patients. Cancer 2017;123(2):319–26.

23. Klemanski DL, Browning KK, Kue J. Survivorship care plan preferences of cancer survivors and health care providers: a systematic review and quality appraisal of the evidence. J Cancer Surviv 2016;10(1):71–86.

24. Cheung WY, Neville BA, Cameron DB, et al. Comparisons of patient and physician expectations for cancer survivorship care. J Clin Oncol 2009;27(15):2489–95.

25. Klabunde CN, Han PK, Earle CC, et al. Physician roles in the cancer-related follow-up care of cancer survivors. Fam Med 2013;45(7):463–74.

26. Potosky AL, Han PK, Rowland J, et al. Differences between primary care physicians' and oncologists' knowledge, attitudes and practices regarding the care of cancer survivors. J Gen Intern Med 2011;26(12):1403–10.

27. Grunfeld E, Levine MN, Julian JA, et al. Randomized trial of long-term follow-up for early-stage breast cancer: a comparison of family physician versus specialist care. J Clin Oncol 2006;24(6):848–55.

28. Smith SM, Allwright S, O'Dowd T. Does sharing care across the primary-specialty interface improve outcomes in chronic disease? A systematic review. Am J Manag Care 2008;14(4):213–24.

29. Salz T, Weinberger M, Ayanian JZ, et al. Variation in use of surveillance colonoscopy among colorectal cancer survivors in the United States. BMC Health Serv Res 2010;10:256.

30. Snyder CF, Frick KD, Peairs KS, et al. Comparing care for breast cancer survivors to non-cancer controls: a five-year longitudinal study. J Gen Intern Med 2009;24(4):469–74.

31. Earle CC, Burstein HJ, Winer EP, et al. Quality of non-breast cancer health maintenance among elderly breast cancer survivors. J Clin Oncol 2003;21(8):1447–51.

32. Snyder CF, Frick KD, Herbert RJ, et al. Comorbid condition care quality in cancer survivors: role of primary care and specialty providers and care coordination. J Cancer Surviv 2015;9(4):641–9.

33. Cheung WY, Neville BA, Earle CC. Associations among cancer survivorship discussions, patient and physician expectations, and receipt of follow-up care. J Clin Oncol 2010;28(15):2577–83.

34. Salz T, Baxi S. Moving survivorship care plans forward: focus on care coordination. Cancer Med 2016;5(7):1717–22.
35. Mayer DK, Nekhlyudov L, Snyder CF, et al. American Society of Clinical Oncology clinical expert statement on cancer survivorship care planning. J Oncol Pract 2014;10(6):345–51.
36. Stricker CT, Jacobs LA, Risendal B, et al. Survivorship care planning after the Institute of Medicine recommendations: how are we faring? J Cancer Surviv 2011;5(4):358–70.
37. Ezendam NP, Nicolaije KA, Kruitwagen RF, et al. Survivorship Care Plans to inform the primary care physician: results from the ROGY care pragmatic cluster randomized controlled trial. J Cancer Surviv 2014;8(4):595–602.
38. Salz T, Oeffinger KC, McCabe MS, et al. Survivorship care plans in research and practice. CA Cancer J Clin 2012;62(2):101–17.
39. Commission on Cancer. Cancer Program Standards: Ensuring Patient-Centered Care. Chicago (IL): American College of Surgeons; 2016.
40. Palmer SC, Stricker CT, Panzer SL, et al. Outcomes and satisfaction after delivery of a breast cancer survivorship care plan: results of a multicenter trial. J Oncol Pract 2015;11(2):e222–9.
41. Mayer DK, Birken SA, Check DK, et al. Summing it up: an integrative review of studies of cancer survivorship care plans (2006-2013). Cancer 2015;121(7): 978–96.
42. Parry C, Kent EE, Forsythe LP, et al. Can't see the forest for the care plan: a call to revisit the context of care planning. J Clin Oncol 2013;31(21):2651–3.
43. Aubin M, Giguere A, Martin M, et al. Interventions to improve continuity of care in the follow-up of patients with cancer. Cochrane Database Syst Rev 2012;(7):CD007672.
44. Grunfeld E, Julian JA, Pond G, et al. Evaluating survivorship care plans: results of a randomized, clinical trial of patients with breast cancer. J Clin Oncol 2011; 29(36):4755–62.
45. Mayer DK, Birken SA, Chen RC. Avoiding implementation errors in cancer survivorship care plan effectiveness studies. J Clin Oncol 2015;33(31):3528–30.
46. Halpern MT, Viswanathan M, Evans TS, et al. Models of cancer survivorship care: overview and summary of current evidence. J Oncol Pract 2015;11(1):e19–27.
47. McCabe MS, Partridge AH, Grunfeld E, et al. Risk-based health care, the cancer survivor, the oncologist, and the primary care physician. Semin Oncol 2013;40(6): 804–12.
48. Szalda D, Ginsberg JP. The adult childhood cancer survivor and the general internist: suggestions for patient and provider education. Ann Intern Med 2014; 160(1):66–7.
49. Nekhlyudov L. Integrating primary care in cancer survivorship programs: models of care for a growing patient population. Oncologist 2014;19(6):579–82.
50. Hong S, Nekhlyudov L, Didwania A, et al. Cancer survivorship care: exploring the role of the general internist. J Gen Intern Med 2009;24(Suppl 2):S495–500.
51. Absolom K, Eiser C, Michel G, et al. Follow-up care for cancer survivors: views of the younger adult. Br J Cancer 2009;101(4):561–7.
52. Blaauwbroek R, Zwart N, Bouma M, et al. The willingness of general practitioners to be involved in the follow-up of adult survivors of childhood cancer. J Cancer Surviv 2007;1(4):292–7.
53. Sisler J, Chaput G, Sussman J, et al. Follow-up after treatment for breast cancer: practical guide to survivorship care for family physicians. Can Fam Physician 2016;62(10):805–11.

Long-Term and Latent Side Effects of Specific Cancer Types

Nana Gegechkori, MD, PhD[a], Lindsay Haines, MD[b],
Jenny J. Lin, MD, MPH[a],*

KEYWORDS

- Cancer survivorship • Side effects • Cancer treatment • Symptom management

KEY POINTS

- Most cancer survivors experience some long-term or latent side effects as a result of cancer treatment.
- Fatigue and mental health issues are very common long-term side effects associated with treatment of many different cancers.
- Clinicians should be aware of these long-term and latent side effects so that they can routinely screen for and treat cancer survivors appropriately.

INTRODUCTION

There are currently more than 15 million cancer survivors in the United States, and it is estimated that with improved treatment and early detection, the number of cancer survivors will increase to more than 20 million by 2026.[1] Many of these survivors experience long-term and latent effects from cancer treatment. Long-term effects are side effects that arise during treatment and may persist over time, whereas latent effects may not appear until many years after treatment completion. This article summarizes the common long-term and latent treatment effects for several highly prevalent cancers.

BREAST CANCER

Breast cancer (BC) is the most common non-skin cancer among women, and there are currently greater than 3.5 million BC survivors in the United States, representing more

Disclosures: None of the authors have any conflicts of interest to disclose.
[a] Division of General Internal Medicine, Icahn School of Medicine at Mount Sinai, One Gustave L. Levy Place, Box 1087, New York, NY 10029, USA; [b] Department of Medicine, Icahn School of Medicine at Mount Sinai, One Gustave L. Levy Place, Box 1087, New York, NY 10029, USA
* Corresponding author.
E-mail address: jenny.lin@mssm.edu

Med Clin N Am 101 (2017) 1053–1073
http://dx.doi.org/10.1016/j.mcna.2017.06.003
0025-7125/17/© 2017 Elsevier Inc. All rights reserved.

medical.theclinics.com

than 40% of female cancer survivors.[1] Most women are diagnosed at early stage, and 5-year survival rate is 89%. Risks for developing long-term side effects after BC treatment are multifactorial and include age at the time of diagnosis, comorbidities, and type, dose, and duration of treatment. Common side effects include lymphedema, cardiotoxicity, fatigue, neuropathy, cognitive dysfunction, endocrine disruptions, infertility, sexual health issues, body image concerns, and mental health issues (**Table 1**).

Lymphedema

Lymphedema is a common complication that occurs in approximately 20% of women following surgery or radiation.[2] Compared with isolated radiation to the breast or chest wall, regional lymph node radiation is associated with an increased risk of lymphedema (22% vs 3%).[3] However, the severity of lymphedema varies, even among patients who receive similar treatment, and can cause mild discomfort or pain to severe swelling and disfiguration and may increase risk for cellulitis.[4] Treatment of lymphedema includes lymphatic drainage massage and use of compression sleeves.

Table 1
Long-term and latent effects of breast cancer treatment

Side Effect	Treatment Type				
	Chemo	HT	IM	RT	Surgery
General					
Fatigue	X	—	—	X	—
Pain	—	—	—	X	X
Weakness	X	—	—	X	X
Cardiac					
Cardiomyopathy	X	—	X	X	—
Thromboembolism	—	X	—	—	—
Endocrine					
Bone loss	—	X	—	—	—
Infertility	X	X	—	—	—
Premature menopause	X	X	—	—	—
Vasomotor symptoms	X	X	—	—	—
Musculoskeletal					
Arthralgia/myalgias	—	X	—	—	—
Lymphedema	—	—	—	X	X
Rotator cuff disease	—	—	—	—	X
Neurologic					
Cognitive dysfunction	X	X	—	—	X
Neuropathy	X	—	—	—	—
Psychosocial (anxiety, body image concerns, depression)	—	X	—	X	X
Pulmonary (pneumonitis)	—	—	—	X	—
Sexual dysfunction (decreased libido, vaginal dryness, dyspareunia)	X	—	—	—	—

Abbreviations: Chemo, chemotherapy; IM, immune modulators (trastuzumab).

Cardiotoxicity

Certain types of radiation and chemotherapy are associated with increased risk of developing cardiovascular complications, and some of these effects may not present until up to 20 years after cancer treatment.[5] Cardiovascular complications can include hypertension, arrhythmias, coronary artery disease, heart failure, valvular disease, thromboembolic disorders, peripheral vascular disease, stroke, pulmonary hypertension, and pericardial complications.[6] Anthracycline-induced dose-dependent cardiotoxicity has been observed in 9% of adult patients, with the highest incidence in the first year after chemotherapy completion.[7] However, there is significant variability among patients in their susceptibility to anthracyclines, and a recent study found an estimated cumulative incidence of 26% for doxorubicin-related heart failure.[8] Older age appears to be a significant risk factor for doxorubicin-related cardiotoxicity even with lower doses.[9] Furthermore, cisplatin can also increase the risk of cardiovascular events even decades after treatment completion.[10]

Studies have also shown cardiotoxicity in up to 30% of BC survivors who have received trastuzumab (for HER2+BC).[11-15] Trastuzumab use in combination with doxorubicin leads to >7-fold increase risk of heart failure.[16] Recent studies suggest that cardiotoxicity associated with trastuzumab progressively increases during the 3 to 5 years after treatment completion and can persist many years.[12,17]

Radiation therapy (RT) is also associated with a variety of cardiovascular complications involving the pericardium, myocardium, valves, coronary arteries, and conduction system. Studies have identified regional perfusion defects in nonsymptomatic BC survivors after RT, and the incidence and extent of perfusion defects are closely related to the volume of left ventricle included in the radiation field.[18] Incidence of radiation-induced cardiotoxicity is estimated to be 10% to 30% 5 to 10 years after treatment.[19]

Last, BC survivors may be at higher risk for thrombus formation. A misbalance between release of von Willebrand factor and production of thrombomodulin and adenosine diphosphatase may lead to increased platelet adherence and thrombus formation in irradiated capillaries and arteries.[18] Adjuvant hormonal therapy (HT) with tamoxifen can also increase risk of venous thromboembolism.[20]

Fatigue

Fatigue is the most common symptom experienced by BC survivors, with prevalence rates ranging from 15% to 30% to 70% to 99%.[21,22] Cancer-related fatigue may remain for years after treatment. Mechanisms for persistent fatigue among cancer survivors are not yet fully understood; several pathways, including chronic inflammation, autonomic imbalance, hypothalamic-pituitary-adrenal-axis dysfunction, and mitochondrial damage, may cause disruption of normal neuronal function and result in fatigue.[23] Physical activity has been shown to improve fatigue symptoms.[24]

Neuropathy

About 58% of survivors develop chemotherapy-induced peripheral neuropathy (CIPN).[25] Docetaxel-related peripheral neuropathy can persist up to 1 to 3 years after treatment completion with significant impairment of quality of life.[26] At least one oncology-related neurologic complication such as neuropathic pain, CIPN, phantom breast pain/syndrome, and cognitive decline was found among 48% of BC survivors.[27]

Cognitive Dysfunction

Impairment of cognitive function, such as problems with concentration, executive function, and memory, are reported in up to 35% of BC survivors after treatment completion.[28] Cognitive impairment is a multifactorial phenomenon and associated with chemotherapy, HT, and anesthesia during surgery. Age, comorbidities, and genetic factors are significantly related to risk for cognitive dysfunction.[29]

Bone Health and Musculoskeletal Issues

Almost 80% of BC survivors experience some degree of bone loss.[30] Long-term HT negatively influences bone mineral density and quality.[31,32] Treatment with aromatase inhibitors (AI) is associated with an almost 5 times higher fracture risk.[33] Current smoking, low body mass index, dementia, and corticosteroid use compound fracture risk associated with AIs.[34] Vertebral fractures unrelated to bone density have also been observed among BC survivors.[35]

 BC survivors may report musculoskeletal issues after surgery, such as decreased shoulder range of motion, rotator cuff disease, adhesive capsulitis, or axillary web syndrome.[36] AIs are also associated with increased incidence of arthralgias and myalgias.[37] Treatment includes physical therapy and use of nonsteroidal inflammatory agents.

Premature Menopause and Infertility

Use of chemotherapeutic agents and adjuvant HT is linked with premature menopause and infertility.[38] Approximately 10% of BC survivors older than 45 experience chemotherapy-induced menopause, and tamoxifen use is associated with decreased fertility among premenopausal cancer survivors.[39,40] Menopausal symptoms such vasomotor hot flashes are observed among 50% to 70% of tamoxifen users. Symptoms are often more severe in younger patients because of the abrupt change in hormonal status.[41]

Sexual Dysfunction

Sexual issues, such as decreased libido, arousal, or lubrication, anorgasmia, and dyspareunia are common complaints among BC survivors usually secondary to side effects from chemotherapy rather than RT or surgery.[42–44] Problems with sexual desire may also be related to complications of RT such as cardiac and respiratory dysfunction or skin fibrosis leading to decrease sensitivity.[45]

Body Image Concerns

Body image changes caused by loss of a breast, lymphedema, hair loss, skin changes from RT, weight gain, or early menopause affect 31% to 67% of BC survivors and appear to be most relevant for younger women.[46] Sexually active survivors are more vulnerable to decreased self-esteem, poorer mental health, and difficulties in relationships with a partner because of body appearance concerns.[42]

Mental Health Issues

Depression and anxiety symptoms affect up to a quarter of BC survivors.[47] Compared with the general female population, BC survivors have a 60% increased risk of developing depression, anxiety, and stress-related disorders within 10 years after cancer diagnosis.[48] Fear of cancer recurrence affects more than half of BC survivors and may increase risk for developing mental health problems.[49] Screening survivors for distress, depression, and/or anxiety is important to allow clinicians to treat and/or refer survivors appropriately.

COLORECTAL CANCER

Colorectal cancer (CRC) is the third most common cancer diagnosed in the United States, and there are currently more than 1.4 million CRC survivors.[1,50] Because of screening efforts, many patients are diagnosed at early stage, and the overall 5-year survival rate is 65% (and 90% for those diagnosed at early stage). The most common treatment is surgical resection, with additional systemic chemotherapy and/or RT used either in the neoadjuvant or adjuvant setting for more advanced-stage CRC. Long-term and latent side effects for CRC survivors include bowel, bladder, or sexual dysfunction, complications related to an ostomy, peripheral neuropathy, and mental health issues (**Table 2**).[51]

Bowel Dysfunction

RT is linked to considerable bowel and anorectal side effects, such as bowel frequency, urgency, fecal incontinence, radiation proctitis, and perianal irritation. Approximately half of CRC survivors have chronic diarrhea, and RT remains an independent risk factor for long-term fecal incontinence.[52–54] Patients who undergo lower anterior resection, as well as those undergoing sphincter-saving surgery, are also more likely to experience bowel dysfunction.[55] Severe bowel dysfunction may also be associated with urinary dysfunction and negatively affects sexual function or satisfaction with sex life.[56]

Bladder Dysfunction

Bladder dysfunction may present as various complaints. Damage to the sacral splanchnic nerves can cause detrusor denervation leading to decreased sensitivity of the bladder. Preoperative RT is also associated with increased risk of difficulty

Table 2
Long-term and latent effects of colorectal cancer treatment

Side Effect	Chemotherapy	Radiation	Surgery
General			
Fatigue	X	X	—
Pain	—	X	X
Weakness	—	—	—
Cardiotoxicity	X	—	—
GI			
Bowel urgency	—	X	X
Chronic diarrhea	—	X	X
Fecal incontinence	—	X	—
Ostomy complications	—	—	X
Genitourinary (difficulty voiding or incontinence)	—	X	X
Neurologic			
Cognitive dysfunction	X	—	—
Neuropathy	X	—	—
Psychosocial (anxiety, distress, depression)	—	X	X
Sexual dysfunction (decreased libido, ED, vaginal dryness, dyspareunia)	—	X	X

with urinary voiding.[56] Primary symptoms are difficulties with bladder emptying, overflow incontinence, and loss of bladder fullness sensation. Long-term incontinence and/or difficulty in bladder emptying occur in approximately one-third of CRC survivors, although others have reported urinary urgency and urge- or stress-related incontinence in up to three-quarters of CRC survivors.[56,57]

Sexual Dysfunction

Treatment-related sexual dysfunction has been reported in more than a third of CRC survivors.[57–60] Sacral plexus damage that can occur with surgery, such as abdominal perineal resection, is associated with erectile dysfunction (ED) and painful intercourse.[53,61] Sexual dysfunction is reported in up to two-thirds of CRC survivors and may be due to lack of libido, ED, or ejaculatory problems in men, vaginal dryness in women, and dyspareunia.[56] Risk factors leading to sexual dysfunction include autonomic nerve damage, presence of a stoma, anastomotic leak, or preoperative radiation, the presence of a stoma, and perioperative blood loss.[59]

Ostomy/Stoma-Related Complications

Approximately 10% of patients undergoing sphincter-saving resections have a temporary ileostomy.[62] Complications associated with ostomies include peristomal skin irritation, leakage, odor, noise from the appliance, emotional and social distress. The presence of an ostomy may also impact CRC survivors' relationships and sexual intimacy.[63]

Neuropathy

CIPN is a potential long-term effect of oxaliplatin, which is often used to treat advanced CRC. Some studies report that about 77% of cancer survivors experience oxaliplatin-induced grade 2 peripheral neuropathy.[64] Mostly large sensory nerves are affected, leading to various types of paresthesias. Symptoms are partially reversible for most patients, although less than 40% recover completely.[65]

Cognitive Dysfunction

Cognitive impairment has been found to range from 36% to 52% among CRC survivors. The main cognitive domains affecting CRC survivors include processing speed, verbal memory, and attention/working memory.[66] Adjuvant chemotherapy may increase cognitive dysfunction in CRC survivors, although the majority will improve after treatment completion.[67]

Other Treatment Effects

Up to a quarter of CRC survivors may experience chronic pain as a direct result of the cancer or treatment, thus dramatically influencing survivors' recovery and rehabilitation.[68] Radiotherapy may also increase fracture risk, particularly for pelvic fractures.[69] Last, incidence of 5-fluorouracil–associated cardiotoxicity can occur in up to 68% of CRC survivors[70] and may include angina-like chest pain, myocardial infarction, arrhythmias, heart failure, cardiogenic shock, and sudden death. A previous history of coronary artery disease and mediastinal radiotherapy is significantly associated with posttreatment cardiotoxicity.[71–73]

HEAD AND NECK CANCER

Head and neck cancer (HNC) survivors make up approximately 3% of the cancer survivor population.[1] Advances in otolaryngological surgical techniques have improved survival in this population, and for those with early stage disease, it is estimated that about 80% to 90% will undergo full remission.[74] Many undergo multimodal treatments, including surgery, RT, and chemotherapy. Common side effects in HNC survivors include musculoskeletal and neuromuscular dysfunction, upper gastrointestinal (GI) dysfunction, lymphedema, sleep apnea, speech defects, oral health issues, as well as mental health issues (**Table 3**).

Musculoskeletal and Neuromuscular Dysfunction

Development of nerve palsies after head and neck surgery is common, particularly spinal accessory nerve palsy after radical neck dissection.[75] This nerve palsy causes shoulder motion dysfunction by reducing innervation to the upper and middle trapezius. One study found that upper limb dysfunction was reported to some extent in 77% of patients.[76] Those with spinal accessory nerve palsy can undergo physical therapy to strengthen the affected shoulder to improve or maintain range of motion in the joint.

Patients may experience cervical dystonia when the cervical plexus and nerve roots are damaged during surgery or when progressive fibrosis to the nerve roots and plexus occur after radiation. Cervical dystonia tends to affect the sternocleidomastoid, scalene, and trapezius muscles and is characterized by repetitive flexion and rotation of the neck and elevation of the shoulder. The cervical dystonia found

Table 3
Long-term and latent effects of head and neck cancer treatment

Side Effect	Treatment Type		
	Chemotherapy	Radiation	Surgery
General			
Fatigue	X	X	—
Pain	—	—	X
Weakness	X	X	—
Musculoskeletal			
Cervical dystonia	—	X	X
Lymphedema	—	X	X
Shoulder dysfunction	—	X	X
Neurologic			
Cognitive dysfunction	X	—	—
Cervical radiculopathy	X	X	X
Neuropathy	X	—	X
Oropharyngeal			
Dental caries	—	X	—
Dysarthria	—	X	X
Dysphagia/esophageal stricture	—	X	X
Reflux disease	—	X	—
Taste disturbance	—	X	—
Trismus	—	X	X
Xerostomia	—	X	X
Psychosocial (anxiety, distress, depression)	X	X	X
Pulmonary (pulmonary fibrosis)	X	X	—

in HNC survivors is often progressive but is more responsive to treatment options aimed at strengthening and stabilizing the cervical musculature. Treatment of cervical dystonia includes neuromuscular and proprioceptive retraining, myofascial release, and restoration of range of motion with physical therapy. Medications such as pregabalin, gabapentin, and duloxetine have also been found to help with neuropathic pain and spasm.[77] Although botulinum toxin (Botox) has been approved by the US Food and Drug Administration for treatment of cervical dystonia, there is little evidence demonstrating the efficacy of Botox in patients with radiation or surgically induced cervical dystonia. Small studies, however, have demonstrated that Botox can be efficacious in alleviating both spasms and neuropathic pain in this population.[78–80]

Trismus, limited jaw range of motion, is common in HNC survivors and results in difficulty with eating, speaking, and oral hygiene. Trismus is seen in 28% of patients 1-year after treatment, with highest rates after 6 months of treatment.[81] Physical therapy can be helpful but may be inadequate. Studies of HNC survivors who underwent RT and subsequently developed trismus found that a jaw motion appliance may slow progression of trismus.[82] Pregabalin, gabapentin, and duloxetine are also helpful in treating spasms and pain associated with trismus. Pentoxifylline may improve jaw opening, and Botox may reduce pain but does not have an effect on jaw opening.[83,84] A combination of therapies should be recommended to patients with trismus to attempt to maximize quality of life.

Upper Gastrointestinal Symptoms

Upper GI side effects, particularly dysphagia, are especially common in those who have undergone RT, affects almost 50% of HNC survivors treated for locoregionally advanced-stage disease, and 7% subsequently develop esophageal or pharyngeal strictures.[85,86] In extreme cases, dysphagia can lead to chronic aspiration and recurrent infections. Although dysphagia cannot be completely reversed, swallowing exercises and biofeedback can help reduce dysphagia, whereas esophageal dilation can help alleviate stricture. Those with chronic dysphagia, aspiration episodes, postprandial cough, weight loss, or recurrent pneumonia should be referred to a speech pathologist for swallowing assessments. Sudden onset dysphagia should be evaluated for new or recurrent disease.

Lymphedema

Lymphedema is a common late effect of both surgery and RT, affecting up to three-quarters of survivors.[87] Lymphedema can cause decreased neck range of motion, hearing loss, decreased quality of life, while the cosmetic changes associated with lymphedema can also cause social anxiety and depression. Manual lymphatic drainage and compression garments are the standard of care for treatment.

Sleep Apnea

Obstructive sleep apnea (OSA) is a common among HNC survivors undergoing radiation and chemotherapy.[88] Both can cause tongue and laryngeal swelling that persists for years, and restricted neck motion from radiation can compromise airway positioning. Surgical reconstruction may also cause airway obstruction. OSA can lead to pulmonary hypertension, arrhythmias, and heart failure. Fatigue associated with OSA can worsen quality of life. Continuous positive airway pressure at night, behavioral therapy, and weight loss may improve symptoms.

Speech Alterations

Speech can be affected to varying degrees in HNC survivors, ranging from hoarseness to dysarthria.[89] Speech therapy can help improve speech. Those who have undergone a tracheostomy can use a valved voice prosthesis to improve intelligibility of speech. Those with palatal issues can have prosthetic obturators created to help improve speech.[90]

Oral Health Issues

Oral health can often be compromised in HNC survivors. Disruption of salivary flow as well as damage to teeth from chemotherapy or emesis can put HNC survivors at increased risk of dental caries.[91] Furthermore, radiotherapy can remove the gingival attachment from teeth and increase risk of periodontitis, thus leading to tooth loss or infection. Severe cases of gingival attachment loss have resulted in osteonecrosis.[92] Xerostomia is also common due to loss of salivary gland tissue. Conscientious oral care and regular visits to the dentist can help prevent these symptoms.

Mental Health Issues

Like all cancer survivors, HNC survivors are prone to increased risk of depression and anxiety. Unlike other cancer survivors, many HNC patients undergo surgical procedures that often dramatically change facial structure and appearance. These changes can cause avoidance of social situations, embarrassment, and shame, and providers should recognize and refer appropriate patients for counseling.

LUNG CANCER

Lung cancer (LC) is the second most common cancer diagnosed in the United States, although LC survivors only comprise 3% of cancer survivors as a result of most patients being diagnosed at a more advanced stage.[1] However, with increased screening for high-risk individuals, it is anticipated that there may be a stage shift so that most LCs will be diagnosed at an early stage.[93] The 5-year survival rate for those diagnosed at early stage is 55%. Most early-stage LC is treated with surgical resection and adjuvant chemotherapy ± RT. Common long-term treatment side effects include impaired pulmonary function, fatigue, neuropathy, and mental health issues (**Table 4**).

Impaired Pulmonary Function

Because of risk factors for LC, such as heavy tobacco use, many LC survivors have decreased pulmonary function before diagnosis, and both surgery and RT can further reduce pulmonary function.[94] Approximately half of LC survivors have persistent dyspnea years after treatment completion.[95,96] In addition, many survivors report a chronic cough that may affect eating, sleeping, and speaking.[97] Cough may also result from radiation pneumonitis in those who received RT.

Fatigue

Fatigue is the most common side effect in LC survivors, affecting more than 50% and up to 90% of survivors.[98,99] Mood disorders, comorbidities, poor functional status, sleep disturbances, and decreased pulmonary function increase the risk for fatigue. Moreover, fatigue symptoms often cluster with mood and sleep disorders, suggesting a possible common inflammatory pathway. Although fatigue is hard to treat, physical activity and exercise may improve symptoms.[100–102] In addition, targeted therapy such as angiogenesis inhibitors or drugs for LC with *ALK* gene mutations may also

Table 4
Long-term and latent effects of lung cancer treatment

Side Effect	Treatment Type			
	Chemo	RT	Surgery	Targeted
General				
Fatigue	X	X	—	X
Pain	—	—	X	—
Weakness	X	X	—	—
Dermatitis	—	—	—	X
Hypertension	—	—	—	X
Neurologic				
Cognitive dysfunction	X	—	—	—
Neuropathy	X	—	—	—
Psychosocial (anxiety, distress, depression)	X	X	X	—
Pulmonary				
Chronic cough	—	X	—	—
Dyspnea	—	X	X	—
Pneumonitis	—	X	—	—

Targeted refers to immunotherapy drugs that target specific gene mutations (eg, *ALK*), angiogenesis inhibitors, or EGFR inhibitors.

cause fatigue, but it is not yet known how long fatigue symptoms may persist given the very recent use of these drugs.

Neuropathy

Treatment with platinum-based chemotherapy agents may cause CIPN in up to 50% of LC survivors and may persist for years after treatment completion.[103,104] Treatment is variably effective and may include tricyclic antidepressants, anticonvulsants (such as gabapentin or pregabalin), or topical agents. One study also found that duloxetine was effective in reducing pain in survivors with CIPN.[105]

Mental Health Issues

Similar to other cancer survivors, LC survivors also experience higher rates of depression and anxiety, and both are associated with higher cancer-specific and overall mortality.[106–108] However, LC survivors also often cope with the stigma of LC being a "self-inflicted" illness because of its strong association with tobacco use; non-smokers in particular describe feeling stigmatized by LC diagnosis.[109–111]

Other Treatment Effects

Targeted immunotherapy with angiogenesis inhibitors may cause hypertension, increased risk for bleeding, or poor wound healing because of their effect on vascular growth. In addition, epidermal growth factor receptor (EGFR) inhibitors are often associated with an acneiform dermatitis that can range from a mild rash and itching to very severe dermatitis affecting most of the body, severe pruritis, and increased risk for skin infections.[112,113]

PROSTATE CANCER

Prostate cancer is the most common non-skin cancer among men in the United States, and prostate cancer survivors comprise more than 20% of all cancer survivors.[1] The 5-year survival rate is greater than 95%, and most prostate cancer survivors die from noncancer causes. The most common modes of treatment of patients with prostate cancer include surgery, RT, hormone therapy, and active surveillance, and each is associated with its own set of side effects. The most common side effects include urinary, sexual, or bowel dysfunction and mental health issues (**Table 5**).

Urinary Dysfunction

After surgery, many survivors experience stress incontinence. Urinary function for these patients generally improves gradually after surgery and reaches stability after 1 year.[114–116] RT can lead to mucositis and edema in the urinary tract, which over time can lead to stricture, overactive bladder, fistulas, hematuria, decreased bladder capacity, weak urinary stream, and urinary retention. For those with postprostatectomy incontinence, a form of stress incontinence, pelvic floor exercises may be beneficial, but evidence of their efficacy is inconclusive.[117,118] Male urethral slings or artificial urinary sphincters can reduce or eliminate stress incontinence in this population.[119] For those with urge incontinence, often in postradiation patients, anticholinergic medications can be helpful. However, given that many prostate cancer survivors are older, these medications should be given with caution. For those with

Table 5
Long-term and latent effects of prostate cancer treatment

Side Effect	Treatment Type		
	Hormonal (ADT)	Radiation	Surgery
General			
Fatigue	X	X	—
Pain	—	X	X
Weakness	X	X	X
Bowel dysfunction			
Fecal urgency/incontinence	—	X	—
Proctitis	—	X	—
Cardiovascular disease	X	—	—
Endocrine			
Bone loss	X	—	—
Metabolic syndrome/diabetes	X	—	—
Vasomotor symptoms	X	—	—
Weight gain/obesity	X	—	—
Psychosocial (anxiety, body image concerns, depression)	X	X	X
Sexual dysfunction (decreased libido, ED)	X	X	X
Urinary dysfunction			
Incontinence	—	X	X
Urethral stricture	—	X	X
Urgency/frequency	—	X	X

difficulty emptying their bladder, alpha-blockers can be tried. In those with postradiation cystitis, hyperbaric oxygen therapy can be useful.[120]

Bowel Dysfunction

Bowel dysfunction is also common, especially in patients who underwent radiation. Acute side effects of RT include bowel irregularity, cramping, and diarrhea. Over time, patients may experience rectal bleeding due to thinning of the rectal mucosa. In severe cases, patients may develop ulcers and rectourethral fistulas. Patients may also develop sphincter dysfunction causing rectal urgency and frequency. Dietary changes and hyperbaric oxygen therapy have been found to help these symptoms.[120] Fortunately, advances in radiation targeting and therapy have decreased the incidence of these issues.

Sexual Dysfunction

Sexual dysfunction affects nearly all prostate cancer survivors at some point. ED is common; those at highest risk for ED are older men and those with preexisting ED. Early penile rehabilitation after prostate cancer surgery can improve sexual function.[121] Penile rehabilitation includes early phosphodiesterase-5 (PDE-5) inhibitor administration to help preserve smooth muscle and improve erectile function through increased tissue perfusion. For those who fail or have contraindications to PDE-5 inhibitors, intraurethral prostaglandin, vacuum erection devices, and penile prosthesis can be tried. Furthermore, although many patients may initially have ED after surgery, some do recover up to 2 to 4 years after surgery.[122] In contrast to postprostatectomy patients who often have rapid onset of ED with varying degrees of improvement over time, those undergoing RT often experience a delayed onset of symptoms, usually 6 to 36 months after treatment.[123] Those receiving androgen deprivation therapy (ADT) also suffer from ED, usually because of decreased libido.

Although there are many physiologic causes for sexual dysfunction after treatment, psychosocial issues also impact sexual functioning. Many prostate cancer survivors suffer from anxiety and depression after treatment, and these issues may affect sexual drive and function.[124–126] Furthermore, partners of prostate cancer survivors also have high rates of anxiety and depression, which may compound a couple's difficulty achieving intimacy after treatment.[127–129] Concerns over physical changes, such as lack of or changes in ejaculate, shortened penis size, or loss of male secondary sexual characteristics, that can occur with certain treatments may also limit a patient's ability to seek sexual intimacy and may create a psychological barrier to attaining their prior sex life.

Tools such as the Sexual Health Inventory for Men can help clinicians screen for difficulties with sexual intimacy to determine who to refer for counseling as well as to initiate pharmacologic interventions. Besides ED itself, other side effects of treatment such as urinary and bowel dysfunction can interfere with sexual intimacy as well.

Mental Health Issues

Like other survivors, prostate cancer survivors experience greater levels of anxiety and depression. Up to 30% of those with prostate cancer experience general distress; 25% have increased anxiety, and 10% have clinically significant depression.[124–126] Although the bulk of studies assessing mental health examined patients within the first year after treatment, over time the level of distress that prostate cancer survivors experience appears to decrease.[130] Routine distress screening is effective and can also help relieve the distress felt by these survivors.[131]

Other Treatment Effects

ADT can increase risk for obesity and diabetes because of its effect on fat and lipid metabolism, as well as possibly increase risk for cardiovascular disease.[132–134] In addition, ADT use has been associated with increased bone loss and higher incidence of osteoporosis and fractures. Men who have received ADT also may experience vasomotor symptoms, such as hot flashes and night sweats. Periodic screening for diabetes, lipid profiles, and bone density are recommended for prostate cancer survivors who have received ADT.

A summary of treatment side effects associated with each of the cancers described is presented in **Table 6**.

FUTURE CONSIDERATIONS/SUMMARY

With improved screening and treatment, the number of cancer survivors in the United States is expected increase by another 5 million in the next decade. Although many cancer survivors, especially those diagnosed at early stage, will outlive their cancer and die of other comorbidities, their cancer treatments may lead to long-term and/or latent side effects. These side effects often have significant impact on survivors' quality of life, morbidity, and overall mortality. Clinicians, both in primary care and oncology, should be aware of these issues so that they can routinely and actively screen for and treat these side effects in cancer survivors.

Table 6
Common long-term and latent treatment side effects by cancer type

Side Effect	Cancer Type				
	Breast	CRC	HNC	Lung	Prostate
Bone loss	X	—	—	—	X
Bowel dysfunction	—	X	—	—	X
Cardiovascular disease	X	X	—	X	X
Cognitive dysfunction	X	X	—	X	—
Dermatitis	—	—	—	X	—
Dysphagia/GERD	—	—	X	—	—
Endocrine disruptions (infertility, metabolic syndrome, vasomotor symptoms)	X	—	—	—	X
Fatigue	X	X	X	X	X
Lymphedema	X	—	X	—	—
Mental health issues (anxiety, depression, body image concerns)	X	X	X	X	X
Musculoskeletal pain	X	—	X	—	—
Neuropathy	—	X	X	X	—
Oral health issues	—	—	X	—	—
Pulmonary dysfunction	X	—	X	X	—
Sexual dysfunction	X	X	—	—	X
Sleep apnea	—	—	X	—	—
Urinary dysfunction	—	X	—	—	X

Abbreviation: GERD, gastroesophageal reflux disease.

REFERENCES

1. Miller KD, Siegel RL, Lin CC, et al. Cancer treatment and survivorship statistics, 2016. CA Cancer J Clin 2016;66(4):271–89.
2. DiSipio T, Rye S, Newman B, et al. Incidence of unilateral arm lymphoedema after breast cancer: a systematic review and meta-analysis. Lancet Oncol 2013; 14(6):500–15.
3. Warren LE, Miller CL, Horick N, et al. The impact of radiation therapy on the risk of lymphedema after treatment for breast cancer: a prospective cohort study. Int J Radiat Oncol Biol Phys 2014;88(3):565–71.
4. International Society of Lymphology. The diagnosis and treatment of peripheral lymphedema: 2013 consensus document of the International Society of Lymphology. Lymphology 2013;46(1):1–11.
5. Okwuosa TM, Anzevino S, Rao R. Cardiovascular disease in cancer survivors. Postgrad Med J 2017;93(1096):82–90.
6. Zamorano JL, Lancellotti P, Rodriguez Munoz D, et al. 2016 ESC position paper on cancer treatments and cardiovascular toxicity developed under the auspices of the ESC committee for practice guidelines: the Task Force for Cancer Treatments and Cardiovascular Toxicity of the European Society of Cardiology (ESC). Eur Heart J 2016;37(36):2768–801.
7. Cardinale D, Colombo A, Bacchiani G, et al. Early detection of anthracycline cardiotoxicity and improvement with heart failure therapy. Circulation 2015; 131(22):1981–8.
8. Bristow MR, Thompson PD, Martin RP, et al. Early anthracycline cardiotoxicity. Am J Med 1978;65(5):823–32.
9. Swain SM, Whaley FS, Ewer MS. Congestive heart failure in patients treated with doxorubicin: a retrospective analysis of three trials. Cancer 2003;97(11): 2869–79.
10. Brouwers EE, Huitema AD, Beijnen JH, et al. Long-term platinum retention after treatment with cisplatin and oxaliplatin. BMC Clin Pharmacol 2008;8:7.
11. Piccart-Gebhart MJ, Procter M, Leyland-Jones B, et al. Trastuzumab after adjuvant chemotherapy in HER2-positive breast cancer. N Engl J Med 2005;353(16): 1659–72.
12. Ewer SM, Ewer MS. Cardiotoxicity profile of trastuzumab. Drug Saf 2008;31(6): 459–67.
13. Joensuu H, Kellokumpu-Lehtinen P-L, Bono P, et al. Adjuvant docetaxel or vinorelbine with or without trastuzumab for breast cancer. N Engl J Med 2006;354(8): 809–20.
14. Smith I, Procter M, Gelber RD, et al. 2-year follow-up of trastuzumab after adjuvant chemotherapy in HER2-positive breast cancer: a randomised controlled trial. Lancet 2007;369(9555):29–36.
15. Slamon DJ, Leyland-Jones B, Shak S, et al. Use of chemotherapy plus a monoclonal antibody against HER2 for metastatic breast cancer that overexpresses HER2. N Engl J Med 2001;344(11):783–92.
16. Pearson EJ, Nair A, Daoud Y, et al. The incidence of cardiomyopathy in BRCA1 and BRCA2 mutation carriers after anthracycline-based adjuvant chemotherapy. Breast Cancer Res Treat 2017;162(1):59–67.
17. Riccio G, Coppola C, Piscopo G, et al. Trastuzumab and target-therapy side effects: is still valid to differentiate anthracycline type I from type II cardiomyopathies? Hum Vaccin Immunother 2016;12(5):1124–31.

18. Stewart FA, Hoving S, Russell NS. Vascular damage as an underlying mechanism of cardiac and cerebral toxicity in irradiated cancer patients. Radiat Res 2010;174(6):865–9.

19. Hong RA, Iimura T, Sumida KN, et al. Cardio-oncology/onco-cardiology. Clin Cardiol 2010;33(12):733–7.

20. Decensi A, Maisonneuve P, Rotmensz N, et al. Effect of tamoxifen on venous thromboembolic events in a breast cancer prevention trial. Circulation 2005; 111(5):650–6.

21. Andrykowski MA, Donovan KA, Laronga C, et al. Prevalence, predictors, and characteristics of off-treatment fatigue in breast cancer survivors. Cancer 2010;116(24):5740–8.

22. Curt GA, Breitbart W, Cella D, et al. Impact of cancer-related fatigue on the lives of patients: new findings from the fatigue coalition. Oncologist 2000;5(5): 353–60.

23. Berger AM, Mooney K, Alvarez-Perez A, et al. Cancer-related fatigue, version 2.2015. J Natl Compr Canc Netw 2015;13(8):1012–39.

24. Canario AC, Cabral PU, de Paiva LC, et al. Physical activity, fatigue and quality of life in breast cancer patients. Rev Assoc Med Bras (1992) 2016;62(1):38–44.

25. Bao T, Basal C, Seluzicki C, et al. Long-term chemotherapy-induced peripheral neuropathy among breast cancer survivors: prevalence, risk factors, and fall risk. Breast Cancer Res Treat 2016;159(2):327–33.

26. Eckhoff L, Knoop A, Jensen MB, et al. Persistence of docetaxel-induced neuropathy and impact on quality of life among breast cancer survivors. Eur J Cancer 2015;51(3):292–300.

27. Pereira S, Fontes F, Sonin T, et al. Neurological complications of breast cancer: a prospective cohort study. Breast 2015;24(5):582–7.

28. Von Ah D, Habermann B, Carpenter JS, et al. Impact of perceived cognitive impairment in breast cancer survivors. Eur J Oncol Nurs 2013;17(2):236–41.

29. Fernandez-de-las-Penas C, Fernandez-Lao C, Cantarero-Villanueva I, et al. Catechol-O-methyltransferase genotype (Val158met) modulates cancer-related fatigue and pain sensitivity in breast cancer survivors. Breast Cancer Res Treat 2012;133(2):405–12.

30. Chen Z, Maricic M, Pettinger M, et al. Osteoporosis and rate of bone loss among postmenopausal survivors of breast cancer. Cancer 2005;104(7):1520–30.

31. Hong AR, Kim JH, Lee KH, et al. Long-term effect of aromatase inhibitors on bone microarchitecture and macroarchitecture in non-osteoporotic postmenopausal women with breast cancer. Osteoporos Int 2017;28(4):1413–22.

32. Wright LE, Harhash AA, Kozlow WM, et al. Aromatase inhibitor-induced bone loss increases the progression of estrogen receptor-negative breast cancer in bone and exacerbates muscle weakness in vivo. Oncotarget 2017;8(5): 8406–19.

33. Villa P, Lassandro AP, Amar ID, et al. Impact of aromatase inhibitor treatment on vertebral morphology and bone mineral density in postmenopausal women with breast cancer. Menopause 2016;23(1):33–9.

34. Schimdt N, Jacob L, Coleman R, et al. The impact of treatment compliance on fracture risk in women with breast cancer treated with aromatase inhibitors in the United Kingdom. Breast Cancer Res Treat 2016;155(1):151–7.

35. Pedersini R, Monteverdi S, Mazziotti G, et al. Morphometric vertebral fractures in breast cancer patients treated with adjuvant aromatase inhibitor therapy: a cross-sectional study. Bone 2017;97:147–52.

36. Stubblefield MD, Keole N. Upper body pain and functional disorders in patients with breast cancer. PM R 2014;6(2):170–83.

37. Barron TI, Cahir C, Sharp L, et al. A nested case-control study of adjuvant hormonal therapy persistence and compliance, and early breast cancer recurrence in women with stage I-III breast cancer. Br J Cancer 2013;109(6):1513–21.

38. Lambertini M, Cinquini M, Moschetti I, et al. Temporary ovarian suppression during chemotherapy to preserve ovarian function and fertility in breast cancer patients: a GRADE approach for evidence evaluation and recommendations by the Italian Association of Medical Oncology. Eur J Cancer 2017;71:25–33.

39. Shandley LM, Spencer JB, Fothergill A, et al. Impact of tamoxifen therapy on fertility in breast cancer survivors. Fertil Steril 2017;107(1):243–52.e245.

40. Dohou J, Mouret-Reynier MA, Kwiatkowski F, et al. A retrospective study on the onset of menopause after chemotherapy: analysis of data extracted from the Jean Perrin comprehensive cancer center database concerning 345 young breast cancer patients diagnosed between 1994 and 2012. Oncology 2017; 92(5):255–63.

41. Stan D, Loprinzi CL, Ruddy KJ. Breast cancer survivorship issues. Hematol Oncol Clin North Am 2013;27(4):805–27, ix.

42. Fobair P, Spiegel D. Concerns about sexuality after breast cancer. Cancer J 2009;15(1):19–26.

43. Gilbert E, Ussher JM, Perz J. Sexuality after breast cancer: a review. Maturitas 2010;66(4):397–407.

44. Ussher JM, Perz J, Gilbert E. Changes to sexual well-being and intimacy after breast cancer. Cancer Nurs 2012;35(6):456–65.

45. Berkey FJ. Managing the adverse effects of radiation therapy. Am Fam Physician 2010;82(4):381–8, 394.

46. Falk Dahl CA, Reinertsen KV, Nesvold IL, et al. A study of body image in long-term breast cancer survivors. Cancer 2010;116(15):3549–57.

47. Zainal NZ, Nik-Jaafar NR, Baharudin A, et al. Prevalence of depression in breast cancer survivors: a systematic review of observational studies. Asian Pac J Cancer Prev 2013;14(4):2649–56.

48. Yang H, Brand JS, Fang F, et al. Time-dependent risk of depression, anxiety, and stress-related disorders in patients with invasive and in situ breast cancer. Int J Cancer 2017;140(4):841–52.

49. Ellegaard MB, Grau C, Zachariae R, et al. Fear of cancer recurrence and unmet needs among breast cancer survivors in the first five years. A cross-sectional study. Acta Oncol 2017;56(2):314–20.

50. Howlader N, Noone AM, Krapcho M, et al. SEER Cancer Statistics Review, 1975-2014, National Cancer Institute. Bethesda (MD). Available at: https://seer.cancer.gov/csr/1975_2014/. Accessed July 24, 2017.

51. Rim SH, Seeff L, Ahmed F, et al. Colorectal cancer incidence in the United States, 1999-2004: an updated analysis of data from the National Program of Cancer Registries and the Surveillance, Epidemiology, and End Results Program. Cancer 2009;115(9):1967–76.

52. Bruheim K, Guren MG, Skovlund E, et al. Late side effects and quality of life after radiotherapy for rectal cancer. Int J Radiat Oncol Biol Phys 2010;76(4):1005–11.

53. Marijnen CA, van de Velde CJ, Putter H, et al. Impact of short-term preoperative radiotherapy on health-related quality of life and sexual functioning in primary rectal cancer: report of a multicenter randomized trial. J Clin Oncol 2005; 23(9):1847–58.

54. Lange MM, Martz JE, Ramdeen B, et al. Long-term results of rectal cancer surgery with a systematical operative approach. Ann Surg Oncol 2013;20(6): 1806–15.
55. Bregendahl S, Emmertsen KJ, Lous J, et al. Bowel dysfunction after low anterior resection with and without neoadjuvant therapy for rectal cancer: a population-based cross-sectional study. Colorectal Dis 2013;15(9):1130–9.
56. Bregendahl S, Emmertsen KJ, Lindegaard JC, et al. Urinary and sexual dysfunction in women after resection with and without preoperative radiotherapy for rectal cancer: a population-based cross-sectional study. Colorectal Dis 2015;17(1):26–37.
57. Lange MM, Maas CP, Marijnen CA, et al. Urinary dysfunction after rectal cancer treatment is mainly caused by surgery. Br J Surg 2008;95(8):1020–8.
58. Peeters KC, van de Velde CJ, Leer JW, et al. Late side effects of short-course preoperative radiotherapy combined with total mesorectal excision for rectal cancer: increased bowel dysfunction in irradiated patients–a Dutch colorectal cancer group study. J Clin Oncol 2005;23(25):6199–206.
59. Lange MM, Marijnen CA, Maas CP, et al. Risk factors for sexual dysfunction after rectal cancer treatment. Eur J Cancer 2009;45(9):1578–88.
60. Pollack J, Holm T, Cedermark B, et al. Late adverse effects of short-course preoperative radiotherapy in rectal cancer. Br J Surg 2006;93(12):1519–25.
61. Havenga K, Maas CP, DeRuiter MC, et al. Avoiding long-term disturbance to bladder and sexual function in pelvic surgery, particularly with rectal cancer. Semin Surg Oncol 2000;18(3):235–43.
62. Kim MJ, Kim YS, Park SC, et al. Risk factors for permanent stoma after rectal cancer surgery with temporary ileostomy. Surgery 2016;159(3):721–7.
63. Dabirian A, Yaghmaei F, Rassouli M, et al. Quality of life in ostomy patients: a qualitative study. Patient Prefer Adherence 2010;5:1–5.
64. Dault R, Rousseau MP, Beaudoin A, et al. Impact of oxaliplatin-induced neuropathy in patients with colorectal cancer: a prospective evaluation at a single institution. Curr Oncol 2016;23(1):e65–9.
65. Beijers AJ, Mols F, Vreugdenhil G. A systematic review on chronic oxaliplatin-induced peripheral neuropathy and the relation with oxaliplatin administration. Support Care Cancer 2014;22(7):1999–2007.
66. Vardy J, Dhillon H, Pond G, et al. Cognitive function and fatigue after diagnosis of colorectal cancer. Ann Oncol 2014;25(12):2404–12.
67. Cruzado JA, López-Santiago S, Martínez-Marín V, et al. Longitudinal study of cognitive dysfunctions induced by adjuvant chemotherapy in colon cancer patients. Support Care Cancer 2014;22(7):1815–23.
68. Brown MR, Ramirez JD, Farquhar-Smith P. Pain in cancer survivors. Br J Pain 2014;8(4):139–53.
69. Baxter NN, Habermann EB, Tepper JE, et al. Risk of pelvic fractures in older women following pelvic irradiation. JAMA 2005;294(20):2587–93.
70. Rezkalla S, Kloner RA, Ensley J, et al. Continuous ambulatory ECG monitoring during fluorouracil therapy: a prospective study. J Clin Oncol 1989;7(4):509–14.
71. Yeh ETH, Bickford CL. Cardiovascular complications of cancer therapy: incidence, pathogenesis, diagnosis, and management. J Am Coll Cardiol 2009; 53(24):2231–47.
72. Jones RL, Ewer MS. Cardiac and cardiovascular toxicity of nonanthracycline anticancer drugs. Expert Rev Anticancer Ther 2006;6(9):1249–69.
73. Saif MW, Shah MM, Shah AR. Fluoropyrimidine-associated cardiotoxicity: revisited. Expert Opin Drug Saf 2009;8(2):191–202.

74. Cohen EE, LaMonte SJ, Erb NL, et al. American Cancer Society head and neck cancer survivorship care guideline. CA Cancer J Clin 2016;66(3):203–39.

75. Erisen L, Basel B, Irdesel J, et al. Shoulder function after accessory nerve-sparing neck dissections. Head Neck 2004;26(11):967–71.

76. Carr SD, Bowyer D, Cox G. Upper limb dysfunction following selective neck dissection: a retrospective questionnaire study. Head Neck 2009;31(6):789–92.

77. Moore RA, Wiffen PJ, Derry S, et al. Gabapentin for chronic neuropathic pain and fibromyalgia in adults. Cochrane Database Syst Rev 2014;(4):CD007938.

78. Stubblefield MD, Levine A, Custodio CM, et al. The role of botulinum toxin type A in the radiation fibrosis syndrome: a preliminary report. Arch Phys Med Rehabil 2008;89(3):417–21.

79. Stubblefield MD, Manfield L, Riedel ER. A preliminary report on the efficacy of a dynamic jaw opening device (dynasplint trismus system) as part of the multi-modal treatment of trismus in patients with head and neck cancer. Arch Phys Med Rehabil 2010;91(8):1278–82.

80. Bach CA, Wagner I, Lachiver X, et al. Botulinum toxin in the treatment of post-radiosurgical neck contracture in head and neck cancer: a novel approach. Eur Ann Otorhinolaryngol Head Neck Dis 2012;129(1):6–10.

81. Pauli N, Johnson J, Finizia C, et al. The incidence of trismus and long-term impact on health-related quality of life in patients with head and neck cancer. Acta Oncol 2013;52(6):1137–45.

82. Tang Y, Shen Q, Wang Y, et al. A randomized prospective study of rehabilitation therapy in the treatment of radiation-induced dysphagia and trismus. Strahlenther Onkol 2011;187(1):39–44.

83. Chua DT, Lo C, Yuen J, et al. A pilot study of pentoxifylline in the treatment of radiation-induced trismus. Am J Clin Oncol 2001;24(4):366–9.

84. Hartl DM, Cohen M, Julieron M, et al. Botulinum toxin for radiation-induced facial pain and trismus. Otolaryngol Head Neck Surg 2008;138(4):459–63.

85. Francis DO, Weymuller EA Jr, Parvathaneni U, et al. Dysphagia, stricture, and pneumonia in head and neck cancer patients: does treatment modality matter? Ann Otol Rhinol Laryngol 2010;119(6):391–7.

86. Wang JJ, Goldsmith TA, Holman AS, et al. Pharyngoesophageal stricture after treatment for head and neck cancer. Head Neck 2012;34(7):967–73.

87. Deng J, Ridner SH, Dietrich MS, et al. Prevalence of secondary lymphedema in patients with head and neck cancer. J Pain Symptom Manage 2012;43(2):244–52.

88. Zhou J, Jolly S. Obstructive sleep apnea and fatigue in head and neck cancer patients. Am J Clin Oncol 2015;38(4):411–4.

89. van der Molen L, van Rossum MA, Jacobi I, et al. Pre- and posttreatment voice and speech outcomes in patients with advanced head and neck cancer treated with chemoradiotherapy: expert listeners' and patient's perception. J Voice 2012;26(5)(664):e625–33.

90. Marunick M, Tselios N. The efficacy of palatal augmentation prostheses for speech and swallowing in patients undergoing glossectomy: a review of the literature. J Prosthet Dent 2004;91(1):67–74.

91. Epstein JB, Thariat J, Bensadoun RJ, et al. Oral complications of cancer and cancer therapy: from cancer treatment to survivorship. CA Cancer J Clin 2012;62(6):400–22.

92. Marques MA, Dib LL. Periodontal changes in patients undergoing radiotherapy. J Periodontol 2004;75(9):1178–87.

93. Heuvelmans MA, Groen HJ, Oudkerk M. Early lung cancer detection by low-dose CT screening: therapeutic implications. Expert Rev Respir Med 2017; 11(2):89–100.

94. Poghosyan H, Sheldon LK, Leveille SG, et al. Health-related quality of life after surgical treatment in patients with non-small cell lung cancer: a systematic review. Lung Cancer 2013;81(1):11–26.

95. Kenny PM, King MT, Viney RC, et al. Quality of life and survival in the 2 years after surgery for non small-cell lung cancer. J Clin Oncol 2008;26(2):233–41.

96. Ozturk A, Sarihan S, Ercan I, et al. Evaluating quality of life and pulmonary function of long-term survivors of non-small cell lung cancer treated with radical or postoperative radiotherapy. Am J Clin Oncol 2009;32(1):65–72.

97. Harle AS, Blackhall FH, Smith JA, et al. Understanding cough and its management in lung cancer. Curr Opin Support Palliat Care 2012;6(2):153–62.

98. Huang X, Zhou W, Zhang Y. Features of fatigue in patients with early-stage non-small cell lung cancer. J Res Med Sci 2015;20(3):268–72.

99. Hung R, Krebs P, Coups EJ, et al. Fatigue and functional impairment in early-stage non-small cell lung cancer survivors. J Pain Symptom Manage 2011; 41(2):426–35.

100. Paramanandam VS, Dunn V. Exercise for the management of cancer-related fatigue in lung cancer: a systematic review. Eur J Cancer Care (Engl) 2015;24(1): 4–14.

101. Lin YY, Rau KM, Lin CC. Longitudinal study on the impact of physical activity on the symptoms of lung cancer survivors. Support Care Cancer 2015;23(12): 3545–53.

102. Crandall K, Maguire R, Campbell A, et al. Exercise intervention for patients surgically treated for non-small cell lung cancer (NSCLC): a systematic review. Surg Oncol 2014;23(1):17–30.

103. Winton T, Livingston R, Johnson D, et al. Vinorelbine plus cisplatin vs. observation in resected non-small-cell lung cancer. N Engl J Med 2005;352(25): 2589–97.

104. Bezjak A, Lee CW, Ding K, et al. Quality-of-life outcomes for adjuvant chemotherapy in early-stage non-small-cell lung cancer: results from a randomized trial, JBR.10. J Clin Oncol 2008;26(31):5052–9.

105. Smith EM, Pang H, Cirrincione C, et al. Effect of duloxetine on pain, function, and quality of life among patients with chemotherapy-induced painful peripheral neuropathy: a randomized clinical trial. JAMA 2013;309(13):1359–67.

106. Hopwood P, Stephens RJ. Depression in patients with lung cancer: prevalence and risk factors derived from quality-of-life data. J Clin Oncol 2000;18(4): 893–903.

107. Vodermaier A, Lucas S, Linden W, et al. Anxiety after diagnosis predicts lung-cancer specific and overall survival in patients with stage III non-small cell lung cancer. A population-based cohort study. J Pain Symptom Manage 2017;53(6):1057–65.

108. Sullivan DR, Forsberg CW, Ganzini L, et al. Longitudinal changes in depression symptoms and survival among patients with lung cancer: a national cohort assessment. J Clin Oncol 2016;34(33):3984–91.

109. Chambers SK, Dunn J, Occhipinti S, et al. A systematic review of the impact of stigma and nihilism on lung cancer outcomes. BMC Cancer 2012;12:184.

110. Chapple A, Ziebland S, McPherson A. Stigma, shame, and blame experienced by patients with lung cancer: qualitative study. BMJ 2004;328(7454):1470.

111. Cataldo JK, Jahan TM, Pongquan VL. Lung cancer stigma, depression, and quality of life among ever and never smokers. Eur J Oncol Nurs 2012;16(3): 264–9.

112. Becker A, van Wijk A, Smit EF, et al. Side-effects of long-term administration of erlotinib in patients with non-small cell lung cancer. J Thorac Oncol 2010;5(9): 1477–80.

113. Bachet JB, Peuvrel L, Bachmeyer C, et al. Folliculitis induced by EGFR inhibitors, preventive and curative efficacy of tetracyclines in the management and incidence rates according to the type of EGFR inhibitor administered: a systematic literature review. Oncologist 2012;17(4):555–68.

114. Sandhu JS, Eastham JA. Factors predicting early return of continence after radical prostatectomy. Curr Urol Rep 2010;11(3):191–7.

115. Skolarus TA, Weizer AZ, Hedgepeth RC, et al. Understanding early functional recovery after robotic prostatectomy. Surg Innov 2012;19(1):5–10.

116. Srivastava A, Peyser A, Gruschow S, et al. Surgical strategies to promote early continence recovery after robotic radical prostatectomy. Arch Esp Urol 2012; 65(5):529–41.

117. Campbell SE, Glazener CM, Hunter KF, et al. Conservative management for postprostatectomy urinary incontinence. Cochrane Database Syst Rev 2012;(1):CD001843.

118. Goode PS, Burgio KL, Johnson TM 2nd, et al. Behavioral therapy with or without biofeedback and pelvic floor electrical stimulation for persistent postprostatectomy incontinence: a randomized controlled trial. JAMA 2011;305(2):151–9.

119. Herschorn S. Update on management of post-prostatectomy incontinence in 2013. Can Urol Assoc J 2013;7(9–10 Suppl 4):S189–91.

120. Hampson NB, Holm JR, Wreford-Brown CE, et al. Prospective assessment of outcomes in 411 patients treated with hyperbaric oxygen for chronic radiation tissue injury. Cancer 2012;118(15):3860–8.

121. Brewer ME, Kim ED. Penile rehabilitation therapy with PDE-V inhibitors following radical prostatectomy: proceed with caution. Available at: https://www.ncbi.nlm. nih.gov/pmc/articles/PMC2648049/pdf/AU2009-852437.pdf. Accessed July 24, 2017.

122. McCullough AR. Rehabilitation of erectile function following radical prostatectomy. Asian J Androl 2008;10(1):61–74.

123. Skolarus TA, Wolf AM, Erb NL, et al. American Cancer Society prostate cancer survivorship care guidelines. CA Cancer J Clin 2014;64(4):225–49.

124. Jayadevappa R, Malkowicz SB, Chhatre S, et al. The burden of depression in prostate cancer. Psychooncology 2012;21(12):1338–45.

125. Korfage IJ, Essink-Bot ML, Janssens AC, et al. Anxiety and depression after prostate cancer diagnosis and treatment: 5-year follow-up. Br J Cancer 2006; 94(8):1093–8.

126. Punnen S, Cowan JE, Dunn LB, et al. A longitudinal study of anxiety, depression and distress as predictors of sexual and urinary quality of life in men with prostate cancer. BJU Int 2013;112(2):E67–75.

127. Tanner T, Galbraith M, Hays L. From a woman's perspective: life as a partner of a prostate cancer survivor. J Midwifery Womens Health 2011;56(2):154–60.

128. Couper J, Bloch S, Love A, et al. Psychosocial adjustment of female partners of men with prostate cancer: a review of the literature. Psychooncology 2006; 15(11):937–53.

129. Heins M, Schellevis F, Rijken M, et al. Partners of cancer patients consult their GPs significantly more often with both somatic and psychosocial problems. Scand J Prim Health Care 2013;31(4):203–8.
130. Carlson LE, Angen M, Cullum J, et al. High levels of untreated distress and fatigue in cancer patients. Br J Cancer 2004;90(12):2297–304.
131. Norris L, Pratt-Chapman M, Noblick JA, et al. Distress, demoralization, and depression in cancer survivorship. Psychiatr Ann 2011;41(9):433–8.
132. Taylor LG, Canfield SE, Du XL. Review of major adverse effects of androgen-deprivation therapy in men with prostate cancer. Cancer 2009;115(11):2388–99.
133. Saylor PJ, Smith MR. Metabolic complications of androgen deprivation therapy for prostate cancer. J Urol 2013;189(1 Suppl):S34–42 [discussion: S43–4].
134. Nguyen PL, Je Y, Schutz FA, et al. Association of androgen deprivation therapy with cardiovascular death in patients with prostate cancer: a meta-analysis of randomized trials. JAMA 2011;306(21):2359–66.

Survivorship Issues in Adolescent and Young Adult Oncology

Linda Overholser, MD, MPH[a],*, Kristin Kilbourn, PhD, MPH[b],
Arthur Liu, MD, PhD[c]

KEYWORDS

- AYA cancer survivorship • Onco-fertility • Risk-based care • Resiliency
- Proactive care • Health promotion

KEY POINTS

- Adolescent and young adult (AYA) cancer survivors face challenges distinct from those in either younger or older age categories.
- Types of cancer seen in the AYA population overlap with pediatric as well as older adult cancers, although outcomes are not the same.
- Fertility and reproductive health issues are especially important and relevant topics for AYA individuals with cancer.
- It is important to understand and anticipate the psychosocial issues that affect AYA individuals with cancer.
- Primary care provider interaction with AYA cancer survivors provides an opportune moment for health promotion.

INTRODUCTION

Of the estimated 15.5 million individuals with a history of cancer alive in the United States as of 2016 estimates, approximately 644,000 are adolescents and young adults (AYAs) living with cancer.[1] With advances in cancer treatment over the last quarter century, there has been an increasing recognition that AYAs face unique challenges when it comes to a cancer diagnosis. Differences exist worldwide in defining the upper and lower age limits of AYAs in the context of oncology clinical care and research[2]; in the United States, the AYA population is generally defined as ages 15 to 39. Despite

Disclosures: The authors have no significant financial disclosures.
[a] Division of General Internal Medicine, University of Colorado School of Medicine, 12631 East 17th Avenue, Mail Stop B180, Aurora, CO 80045, USA; [b] Department of Psychology, College of Liberal Arts and Sciences, University of Colorado Denver, 1200 Larimer Street, NC 5002-M, PO Box 173364, Denver, CO 80017, USA; [c] Department of Radiation Oncology, University of Colorado School of Medicine, 1665 Aurora Ct, MS F706 Aurora, CO 80045, USA
* Corresponding author.
E-mail address: linda.overholser@ucdenver.edu

Med Clin N Am 101 (2017) 1075–1084
http://dx.doi.org/10.1016/j.mcna.2017.06.002
0025-7125/17/© 2017 Elsevier Inc. All rights reserved.

medical.theclinics.com

the slight disparity in these age ranges, AYA oncology has evolved into a distinct area of study for a variety of reasons. Although bridging the life phases of late childhood and early adulthood, care for AYA individuals often involves transitions in care settings because these patients may begin treatment in a pediatric setting, but continued treatment and/or follow-up often occurs in adult care settings. In addition, the developmental phases that define the young cancer survivor are often marked by important life events, such as graduations, new careers, marriages, and starting families. These factors can impact cancer care all the way from diagnosis through long-term survivorship. Issues around access to care, treatment regimens, and availability of clinical trials, fertility concerns, psychosocial issues, and health behaviors as risk factors for future morbidity must be considered even long after active cancer treatments are completed. Although cancer survivorship is being recognized as a phase of the cancer continuum requiring attention to specific health and psychosocial matters, this takes on special meaning for a population of individuals who are simultaneously navigating changes in education, employment, insurance, family planning, relationships, and physical and social development.

Epidemiology

Cancer survival rates for AYAs have improved over the last 40 years; however, this trend has not kept pace with similar improvements in survival for either younger or older age groups.[3–5] This lag in survival has not always been the case, and up until the last quarter of the twentieth century, the AYA population had higher survival rates that their younger or older counterparts.[4] Recognition of this disparity in survival rates is part of the reason that AYA oncology came to exist as a focus of study and clinical care. The differences between AYA survival and those who were diagnosed at a younger age may be explained in part by the fact that AYAs are less likely to get treated in pediatric cancer settings where treatment regimens may be more aggressive and clinical trials more likely available,[6–8] although there may also be differences in tumor biology.

Cancer is a significant health issue for AYAs, because it remains the leading cause of disease-related death in this age group.[9] From 2002 to 2006, the relative 5-year survival rate for AYA cancers was estimated to be 82.5%.[4] This rate is similar to 5-year survival rates noted in the under 15 age group (82.0%) and better than the over 40 age group (65.9%). There is some recent evidence suggesting the survival trends for adolescents may be catching up to the pediatric cancer population.[10] AYA patients with cancer are less likely to be enrolled in clinical trials.[11]

The types of cancer seen in the AYA population as a group are distinct[9] because they overlap on each end of the spectrum with cancers seen in both the pediatric and the adult populations, although treatment outcomes may differ.[4,12] In this age group for asymptomatic individuals with no previous cancer history and with no increased risk based on hereditary predisposition or family history, the only cancer screening recommended in general practice would be cervical cancer screening in women,[13] such that AYA cancers would not typically be picked up by screening, which is one difference from cancers diagnosed in older populations. Even within the AYA cohort, the prevalence of certain cancers changes based on age of diagnosis such that in younger AYAs (15–24 years) there is a higher prevalence of "pediatric" cancers (leukemia, lymphoma), whereas by the time an individual ages into the older AYA cohort (ages 25–39), breast and colon cancer become more prevalent.[9]

Access to Care

It is known from studies with the childhood cancer survivor population (which includes adolescents) that most individuals treated at pediatric cancer centers are generally followed up as adults in the community primary care setting, away from where their original cancer treatment was provided.[14,15] Seeking care in such a setting decreases the likelihood of receiving survivorship focused care[14,15] and surveillance for late effects,[16] with a greater likelihood of receiving what has been described as "illness-driven" care.[17] This type of care is driven more by acute, episodic symptom management rather than a proactive approach to surveillance for late and long-term effects and discussion of strategies to maintain wellness.[17] There are numerous barriers cited to achieving successful transition from the pediatric oncology setting to the adult primary care setting, including provider, caregiver/family, provider, as well as systemic barriers.[18] Interestingly, in a large observational study of the health status of AYA survivors, despite no differences in insurance or having a personal health provider, survivors report a higher prevalence of not being able to see a medical provider because of cost.[19] Explanations for this may be related to the overall higher cost of cancer-related care (ie, copayments, medications, and so forth) or overall lower income levels, which may be an effect of interruptions in education or employment.[19]

The age range characteristic of AYAs is a time when individuals even without a cancer history are more likely to not have health insurance.[20] Moreover, if children and younger adolescents are covered by safety net insurance programs, loss of that safety net upon entering adulthood puts them at risk of being unable to access care and/or increased financial risk.[20] For AYAs with a diagnosis of cancer, lack of health insurance can adversely affect long-term survival.[21] Learning to navigate the health care system and being able to access and maintain health insurance coverage, which may or may not come from an employer, is a new skill that must be acquired by emerging adults. There is some evidence that more 18- to 25-year-old AYA survivors reported having health insurance after the implementation of the Patient Protection and Affordable Care Act in 2010[22]; this was likely attributable to the dependent care provisions because similar changes were not seen in the 26- to 29-year-old age group.

In addition to financial and insurance-related issues, there are other significant barriers to AYAs accessing quality medical care, and one can learn here from examples in both the childhood and the adult cancer populations (**Box 1**). Competing life

---

Box 1
Barriers for adolescent and young adult cancer survivors in receiving appropriate follow-up care

Practical

Financial/cost

Lack of or inadequate insurance

Competing life demands/responsibilities (work, childcare, relocation)

Health care system related

Lack of provider recommendation for long-term follow-up

Need for provider survivorship education

Lack of resources for survivorship focused care

Psychosocial/health related

Desire to put/keep cancer history in past

PTSD symptoms/anxiety

Lack of perceived need for follow-up/lack of symptoms

demands, such as childcare responsibilities, and work and school responsibilities, as well as a lack of recommendations on the part of providers and a lack of perceived need for follow-up when not having symptoms, may all play a role.[23] Some survivors may express a desire to move on from their cancer history and keep it in the past, which leads to an avoidance of survivorship care.

To complicate these potential barriers around access to care on the patient side is the role of the provider. In particular, primary care providers have expressed an interest to care for adult survivors of childhood and adolescent cancer, although there has not been consensus of the best way to provide follow-up care.[24] Perceived lack of knowledge about survivorship care and a lack of clarity in roles following active cancer treatment have recently been identified as a barrier to transition from oncology to primary care.[25,26]

Psychosocial Concerns

Research has demonstrated that psychosocial concerns are common in cancer survivors, but there are special considerations for AYA individuals owing to their developmental stages and the normal life changes occurring during this time. A recent systematic review indicates that both achieving educational goals and maintaining employment are more difficult for AYAs with cancer.[27] An important factor to consider is how challenges in educational and workplace settings could potentially lead to further psychosocial distress, given that these settings impact self-esteem and self-worth and also serve as important venues for social interaction with peers.[27]

Anxiety and depression as well as fear of recurrence are commonly studied adverse late and long-term effects of cancer treatment. Being in the AYA age group with a cancer diagnosis may predispose individuals to more depression and anxiety[28] as well as a higher level of fear of recurrence and overall quality-of-life issues.[29,30] However, the range of psychosocial side effects is not limited to anxiety and depression. Individuals may also experience symptoms of posttraumatic stress from their treatments,[31] although they may not be recognized as such. The quality of family support may play a crucial role here, because studies have shown that of a sample of adolescent survivors with posttraumatic stress disorder (PTSD), about 75%, came from families with significant dysfunction.[32,33] Recognizing survivorship-related PTSD in young cancer survivors is important because it can impact health behaviors adversely, such as avoiding medical visits and adoption of behaviors that are risky to health.[34] The presence of comorbidities may also increase the likelihood of need for mental health support.[35]

For all of the discussion around the risks of a poor psychosocial outcomes related to past cancer treatment, there are also potential positive benefits. Recent studies have examined resiliency, posttraumatic growth, and benefit finding as positive outcomes of the cancer experience.[36–38] Some AYA cancer survivors describe positive changes in self, relationships, and life goals as a result of the traumatic experience of cancer and cancer therapy.[36]

Reproductive Health Issues

Fertility

Fertility concerns and fertility preservation rank high on the list of concerns for AYA cancer survivors. Oncofertility has now emerged as a distinct clinical specialty and has been reported as a "signature area of needed care" for these individuals.[39]

Treatment of cancer can affect fertility in both men and women. For example, alkylating agents are known to have adverse effects on spermatogenesis in men and on ovarian function in women. Radiation can affect fertility in 2 ways: either direct effects on gonadal function if in the field of radiation, or secondary effects on reproductive hormones produced by the pituitary axis if cranial radiation is received (but generally these secondary hormonal effects are seen with higher doses of radiation, for example, >40 Gy).[40] Surgery may involve reproductive organs directly, or through scarring. Hormonal changes such as premature ovarian failure in women can predispose to physical changes that negatively impact intimacy and libido. For those trying to conceive, estimates show that just over half of AYA cancer survivors are successful.[39]

Pregnancy

For women who do become pregnant, cancer treatment can result in increased risks for carrying a pregnancy to term. Both surgery and pelvic radiation that affect the uterus, cervix, or birth canal can leave women with significant scarring or anatomic derangements. For women at risk for cardiomyopathy, pregnancy can precipitate cardiac decompensation.

MANAGEMENT GOALS

A key to caring for AYA individuals with a history of cancer is to be aware of their unique needs and concerns. Because fertility is such a prevalent and unique concern in the AYA population, discussion of the effects of cancer and its treatment on fertility are recommended to be discussed early on by treating providers, ideally before cancer treatment is started.[41,42] It is important to assess for anticipated late and long-term effects and provide information to patients about their risks as well as providing appropriate referrals if needed. Even after cancer treatment is completed, the primary care provider can play a big role in providing support and guidance.

Adherence to Current Survivorship Recommendations

The primary goal of follow-up for individuals who have been treated for cancer as an AYA should be to provide risk-based care,[17] that is, to assess current health status, support health behaviors, and make recommendations tailored to individuals based on past cancer diagnoses and treatment as risk factors themselves for future disease. Current guidelines for risk-based surveillance of late and long-term effects are available for adult survivors of childhood cancer (available at http://survivorshipguidelines.org)[43] as well as for the AYA population.[42] These 2 resources apply to individuals in the AYA category, although there are slight differences.[44] Despite such guidance, a recent retrospective study of AYA cancer survivors confirmed not only that adherence is suboptimal,[45] but also that this occurs even despite having a source of follow-up focused on survivorship care, and that adherence rates actually decrease as AYA survivors age. One of the major goals for follow-up of individuals who have been treated for cancer as an AYA should be to review future risks with survivors, currently available guidelines for monitoring of these risks, and strategies to help reduce not only risks for morbidity but also for comorbid conditions.

PHARMACOLOGIC STRATEGIES

There are limited data on the use of pharmacologic strategies to manage symptoms and risks in AYA cancer survivors any differently than in individuals without a cancer history. For example, anxiety and depression can be managed with a wide variety of pharmacologic options, including serotonin specific reuptake inhibitors, tricyclic antidepressants, serotonin-norepinephrine reuptake inhibitors, and benzodiazepines. The exceptions may be agents that could be used for risk reduction in certain individuals who face a higher risk of secondary cancer due to previous treatment exposures as cancer survivors, or due to genetic predisposition by a strong family history or by detection of known high-risk mutations. Examples of areas being studied include the following:

- Low-dose tamoxifen to reduce the risk of breast cancer in women exposed to chest radiation as part of their treatment is being investigated (ClinicalTrials. gov identifier: NCT01196936).
- Aspirin to reduce the risk of colon cancer for individuals with hereditary cancer syndromes that may affect younger individuals.[46]

Other potential scenarios that may include a pharmacologic approach for the management of treatment related late effects include the following:

- Use of reproductive hormones may help manage menopausal symptoms and reduce risk of osteoporosis in women facing premature ovarian failure if not contraindicated in the setting of hormone-sensitive cancers of the breast or reproductive organs. In some women for whom estrogen or progesterone may be contraindicated, alternative therapies could be considered, as for any menopausal woman who has this contraindication.
- For individuals who have had cranial radiation, who have been on growth hormone (GH) replacement therapy, or who are having other suggestive symptoms of GH deficiency, consideration may be given to GH therapy. However, the use of GH therapy is adults is controversial.[47] If therapy is considered, then referral to an adult endocrinologist would be most helpful.
- Use of agents to help with assisted reproduction would be guided by a specialist in Reproductive Medicine.
- Significant anxiety, depression, and/or PTSD may require medication to manage symptoms and may be done so in conjunction with psychotherapy.

NONPHARMACOLOGIC STRATEGIES
Health Promotion

A major task of primary care providers is to provide counseling to promote health. Given that AYAs with cancer face a disproportionately higher risk of future morbidity from their cancer and its treatment, health promotion becomes especially meaningful. In a large observational study of behavioral risk factors for disease, AYA cancer survivors overall self-report higher rates of current smoking, obesity, and physical inactivity.[19] Having any risk factors for cardiovascular disease (CVD), a leading cause of adult morbidity, significantly increased risk of both developing CVD compared with age-matched controls without cancer, and also increased risk of premature mortality from CVD.[48] Health behaviors such as smoking and physical activity are modifiable, and the survivorship phase of care for these individuals would be an ideal opportunity to provide education.

For women with exposures that included either pelvic irradiation or alkylating agent chemotherapy, guidance is available for prospective screening of premature ovarian insufficiency.[49]

Psychosocial Support

All cancer survivors should be screened for distress before, during, and after cancer treatment. Research has shown that cancer survivors may experience elevated levels of distress many years after the completion of treatment.[50] Ultimately, screening and subsequent treatment of elevated depression and/or anxiety will fall to the hands of the adult primary care provider. Being able to anticipate the anxiety and uncertainty that many AYA survivors face, compounded by specific milestones that also lead to increased stress and life disruption, can go a long way to relieving distress.

Referrals

Even with appropriate knowledge about the physical late and long-term effects of cancer, one of the most important roles a primary care provider can play is that of a care coordinator. Referrals to specialists such as Reproductive Medicine, Endocrinology, Physical Therapy, or Cardiology may be necessary.

EVALUATION, ADJUSTMENT, AND RECURRENCE

Monitoring for late and long-term effects, conducting psychosocial assessment and support, providing ongoing preventive care and comorbid disease management as well as surveillance for cancer recurrence require thoughtful coordination between the treating oncology team, the primary care provider, and any involved specialty care providers. Such coordination of care is not unique to the AYA population, but there may be specific needs identified. For many longer-term AYA survivors, they no longer undergo routine surveillance for recurrence of their initial diagnosis. For those survivors who have second cancers not considered to be late effects of previous treatment or suggestive family histories, genetic counseling may be prudent to identify hereditary cancer syndromes if not previously identified. For those AYA survivors with recurrent pediatric cancers, consultation with a pediatric oncologist should be considered.

SUMMARY

The transition into early adulthood is often a stressful period given the number of stressful life changes that are often experienced, such as educational transitions, starting new careers, marriage, and parenthood. Not surprisingly, a diagnosis of cancer during this developmental period can be particularly disruptive. Adult primary care providers will need to be prepared to care for AYA survivors in a proactive way. As more is learned about the unique characteristics of this population of cancer survivors and about the late and long-term effects of cancer therapy to a degree similar to what has been done with the childhood cancer survivor population, one will be able to make recommendations to support tailored, risk-based care. What was once considered impossible for some AYA survivors in regards to fertility is now possible; the future is likely to bring to light new strategies that will continue such advances. The promise of personalized medicine may help to understand who in this population may be most susceptible to known late and long-term effects of therapy. This potential holds true as well for understudied populations of cancer survivors in general, let alone AYA cancer survivors, because currently there is evidence that is not well generalized to minority and underrepresented individuals.

Multimorbidity is becoming more common in primary care. With ongoing advances in treatment and the generally longer lifespan of AYA individuals with cancer, it is likely soon to become the norm. It will require a shift in the way of thinking about cancer as well as how we support AYA individuals with chronic diseases (because cancer can in many cases be considered a chronic disease). Survivorship teaches us that the experience of cancer as well as its treatment in many ways can be considered a risk factor for disease. As we build the evidence base in AYA survivorship we can learn strategies to better manage symptoms and control the burden of cancer.

REFERENCES

1. Miller KD, Siegel RL, Lin CC, et al. Cancer treatment and survivorship statistics, 2016. CA Cancer J Clin 2016;66(4):271–89.
2. What should the age range be for AYA oncology? J Adolesc Young Adult Oncol 2011;1(1):3–10.
3. Lewis DR, Seibel NL, Smith AW, et al. Adolescent and young adult cancer survival. J Natl Cancer Inst Monogr 2014;2014(49):228–35.
4. Keegan THM, Ries LAG, Barr RD, et al. Comparison of cancer survival trends in the United States of adolescents and young adults with those in children and older adults. Cancer 2016;122(7):1009–16.
5. Bleyer A. Latest estimates of survival rates of the 24 most common cancers in adolescent and young adult Americans. J Adolesc Young Adult Oncol 2011; 1(1):37–42.
6. Albritton KH, Wiggins CH, Nelson HE, et al. Site of oncologic specialty care for older adolescents in Utah. J Clin Oncol 2007;25(29):4616–21.
7. Howell DL, Ward KC, Austin HD, et al. Access to pediatric cancer care by age, race, and diagnosis, and outcomes of cancer treatment in pediatric and adolescent patients in the state of Georgia. J Clin Oncol 2007;25(29):4610–5.
8. Pollock BH. Where adolescents and young adults with cancer receive their care: does it matter? J Clin Oncol 2007;25(29):4522–3.
9. NationalCancerInstitute. A snapshot of adolescent and young adult cancers. 2014. Available at: https://www.cancer.gov/research/progress/snapshots/adolescent-young-adult. Accessed July 30, 2017.
10. Smith MA, Altekruse SF, Adamson PC, et al. Declining childhood and adolescent cancer mortality. Cancer 2014;120(16):2497–506.
11. Roth ME, O'Mara AM, Seibel NL, et al. Low enrollment of adolescents and young adults onto cancer trials: insights from the community clinical oncology program. J Oncol Pract 2016;12(4):e388–95.
12. Bleyer A, O'Leary M, Barr R, et al. Cancer epidemiology in older adolescents and young adults 15 to 29 years of age, including SEER incidence and survival: 1975-2000. Bethesda (MD): National Institutes of Health; 2006. NIH Pub. No. 06-5767.
13. UnitedStatesPreventiveServicesTaskForce. United States Preventive Services Task Force Published Recommendations. 2017. Available at: https://www.uspreventiveservicestaskforce.org/BrowseRec/Index. Accessed July 30, 2017.
14. Nathan PC, Greenberg ML, Ness KK, et al. Medical care in long-term survivors of childhood cancer: a report from the childhood cancer survivor study. J Clin Oncol 2008;26(27):4401–9.
15. Oeffinger KC, Mertens AC, Hudson MM, et al. Health care of young adult survivors of childhood cancer: a report from the childhood cancer survivor study. Ann Fam Med 2004;2(1):61–70.
16. Cox CL, Hudson MM, Mertens A, et al. Medical screening participation in the childhood cancer survivor study. Arch Intern Med 2009;169(5):454–62.
17. Oeffinger KC. Longitudinal risk-based health care for adult survivors of childhood cancer. Curr Probl Cancer 2003;27(3):143–67.
18. Freyer DR. Transition of care for young adult survivors of childhood and adolescent cancer: rationale and approaches. J Clin Oncol 2010;28(32):4810–8.
19. Tai E, Buchanan N, Townsend J, et al. Health status of adolescent and young adult cancer survivors. Cancer 2012;118(19):4884–91.

20. Adams SH, Newacheck PW, Park MJ, et al. Health insurance across vulnerable ages: patterns and disparities from adolescence to the early 30s. Pediatrics 2007;119(5):e1033–9.

21. Keegan THM, DeRouen MC, Parsons HM, et al. Impact of treatment and insurance on socioeconomic disparities in survival after adolescent and young adult hodgkin lymphoma: a population-based study. Cancer Epidemiol Biomarkers Prev 2016;25(2):264–73.

22. Parsons HM, Schmidt S, Tenner LL, et al. Early impact of the patient protection and affordable care act on insurance among young adults with cancer: analysis of the dependent insurance provision. Cancer 2016;122(11):1766–73.

23. Smits-Seemann RR, Kaul S, Zamora ER, et al. Barriers to follow-up care among survivors of adolescent and young adult cancer. J Cancer Surviv 2017;11(1):126–32.

24. Potosky AL, Han PKJ, Rowland J, et al. Differences between primary care physicians' and oncologists' knowledge, attitudes and practices regarding the care of cancer survivors. J Gen Intern Med 2011;26(12):1403–10.

25. Suh E, Daugherty CK, Wroblewski K, et al. General internists' preferences and knowledge about the care of adult survivors of childhood cancer: a cross-sectional survey. Ann Intern Med 2014;160(1):11–7.

26. Grunfeld E, Earle CC. The interface between primary and oncology specialty care: treatment through survivorship. J Natl Cancer Inst Monogr 2010;2010(40):25–30.

27. Warner EL, Kent EE, Trevino KM, et al. Social well-being among adolescents and young adults with cancer: a systematic review. Cancer 2016;122(7):1029–37.

28. Lang MJ, David V, Giese-Davis J. The age conundrum: a scoping review of younger age or adolescent and young adult as a risk factor for clinical distress, depression, or anxiety in cancer. J Adolesc Young Adult Oncol 2015;4(4):157–73.

29. Champion VL, Wagner LI, Monahan PO, et al. Comparison of younger and older breast cancer survivors and age-matched controls on specific and overall QoL domains. Cancer 2014;120(15):2237–46.

30. Lebel S, Beattie S, Arès I, et al. Young and worried: age and fear of recurrence in breast cancer survivors. Health Psychol 2013;32(6):695–705.

31. Kwak M, Zebrack BJ, Meeske KA, et al. Prevalence and predictors of post-traumatic stress symptoms in adolescent and young adult cancer survivors: a 1-year follow-up study. Psychooncology 2013;22(8):1798–806.

32. Ozono S, Saeki T, Mantani T, et al. Psychological distress related to patterns of family functioning among Japanese childhood cancer survivors and their parents. Psychooncology 2010;19(5):545–52.

33. Alderfer MA, Navsaria N, Kazak AE. Family functioning and posttraumatic stress disorder in adolescent survivors of childhood cancer. J Fam Psychol 2009;23(5):717–25.

34. Rourke MT, Stuber ML, Hobbie WL, et al. Posttraumatic stress disorder: Understanding the psychosocial impact of surviving childhood cancer into young adulthood. J Pediatr Oncol Nurs 1999;16(3):126–35.

35. Wu X-C, Prasad PK, Landry I, et al. Impact of the AYA HOPE comorbidity index on assessing health care service needs and health status among adolescents and young adults with cancer. Cancer Epidemiol Biomarkers Prev 2015;24(12):1844–9.

36. Barakat LP, Alderfer MA, Kazak AE. Posttraumatic growth in adolescent survivors of cancer and their mothers and fathers. J Pediatr Psychol 2006;31(4):413–9.

37. Zebrack BJ, Stuber ML, Meeske KA, et al. Perceived positive impact of cancer among long-term survivors of childhood cancer: a report from the childhood cancer survivor study. Psychooncology 2012;21(6):630–9.

38. Michel G, Taylor N, Absolom K, et al. Benefit finding in survivors of childhood cancer and their parents: further empirical support for the Benefit Finding Scale for Children. Child Care Health Dev 2010;36(1):123–9.

39. Nass SJ, Beaupin LK, Demark-Wahnefried W, et al. Identifying and addressing the needs of adolescents and young adults with cancer: summary of an institute of medicine workshop. Oncologist 2015;20(2):186–95.

40. Green DM, Kawashima T, Stovall M, et al. Fertility of female survivors of childhood cancer: a report from the childhood cancer survivor study. J Clin Oncol 2009; 27(16):2677–85.

41. Loren AW, Mangu PB, Beck LN, et al. Fertility preservation for patients with cancer: American Society of Clinical Oncology clinical practice guideline update. J Clin Oncol 2013;31(19):2500–10.

42. Coccia PF, Pappo AS, Altman J, et al. Adolescent and young adult oncology, version 2.2014. J Natl Compr Canc Netw 2014;12(1):21–32.

43. Landier W, Bhatia S, Eshelman DA, et al. Development of risk-based guidelines for pediatric cancer survivors: the Children's Oncology Group long-term follow-up guidelines from the Children's Oncology Group late effects committee and nursing discipline. J Clin Oncol 2004;22(24):4979–90.

44. Barthel EM, Spencer K, Banco D, et al. Is the adolescent and young adult cancer survivor at risk for late effects? It depends on where you look. J Adolesc Young Adult Oncol 2016;5(2):159–73.

45. Reppucci ML, Schleien CL, Fish JD. Looking for trouble: adherence to late-effects surveillance among childhood cancer survivors. Pediatr Blood Cancer 2017;64(2):353–7.

46. Burn J, Gerdes A-M, Macrae F, et al. Long-term effect of aspirin on cancer risk in carriers of hereditary colorectal cancer: an analysis from the CAPP2 randomised controlled trial. Lancet 2011;378(9809):2081–7.

47. Frohman LA. Controversy about treatment of growth hormone-deficient adults: a commentary. Ann Intern Med 2002;137(3):202–4.

48. Chao C, Xu L, Bhatia S, et al. Cardiovascular disease risk profiles in survivors of adolescent and young adult (AYA) cancer: the Kaiser Permanente AYA Cancer Survivors Study. J Clin Oncol 2016;34(14):1626–33.

49. van Dorp W, Mulder RL, Kremer LCM, et al. Recommendations for premature ovarian insufficiency surveillance for female survivors of childhood, adolescent, and young adult cancer: a report from the international late effects of childhood cancer guideline harmonization group in collaboration with the PanCareSurFup consortium. J Clin Oncol 2016;34(28):3440–50.

50. Stanton AL. Psychosocial concerns and interventions for cancer survivors. J Clin Oncol 2006;24(32):5132–7.

Cancer-Related Fatigue in Cancer Survivorship

Chidinma C. Ebede, MD, Yongchang Jang, BS, Carmen P. Escalante, MD*

KEYWORDS

- Cancer-related fatigue • Cancer survivors • Screening • Exercise
- Cognitive behavioral therapy • Psycho-educational therapy • Yoga
- Psychostimulants

KEY POINTS

- Cancer-related fatigue (CRF) is a distressing, persistent, subjective sense of physical, emotional, and/or cognitive tiredness or exhaustion related to cancer or cancer treatment that is not proportional to recent activity and that significantly interferes with usual functioning.
- Screening should be performed at the time of the cancer diagnosis, throughout cancer treatment, and following completion of the essential cancer treatment. A fatigue scoring scale (mild-severe) can be used to evaluate fatigue in cancer survivors. Cancer survivors with moderate to severe CRF require an additional detailed evaluation.
- The general approach to CRF management includes education, counseling, and other strategies. This approach should be used for survivors at all fatigue levels.
- Nonpharmacologic interventions include psychosocial interventions, exercise, yoga, physically based therapy, dietary management, and sleep therapy. Cognitive behavioral therapy, psychoeducational therapy, yoga, and exercise have the most supporting evidence for CRF management (category 1).
- The psychostimulant, methylphenidate, is a pharmacologic intervention that may be considered in CRF. It does not have category 1 supporting evidence and is not US Food and Drug Administration approved for CRF. Antidepressants may also benefit cancer survivors when CRF and depression are both present. Corticosteroids are usually limited to patients with cancer with advanced disease.

INTRODUCTION

Fatigue is perceived as one of the most common and distressing adverse effects of cancer and cancer therapy.[1] The National Comprehensive Cancer Network (NCCN) defines cancer-related fatigue (CRF) as a distressing, persistent, subjective sense of

The authors have nothing to disclose.
Department of General Internal Medicine, The University of Texas M.D. Anderson Cancer Center, 1400 Pressler Street, Unit 1465, Houston, TX 77030-4008, USA
* Corresponding author.
E-mail address: cescalan@mdanderson.org

medical.theclinics.com

physical, emotional, and/or cognitive tiredness or exhaustion related to cancer or cancer treatment that is not proportional to recent activity and interferes with usual functioning.[2] Cancer survivors are characterized as individuals who have a diagnosis of cancer from the time of diagnosis until death.[3]

The general overall predominance of CRF is approximately 48%, despite the fact that it is higher in certain malignancies (eg, pancreatic, breast, lymphoma) and during treatment.[4] Studies report 58% to 94% of patients with breast cancer experience CRF during treatment and 56% to 95% have CRF following adjuvant chemotherapy.[4]

Before cancer treatment, fatigue may be present; however, it generally increases during radiotherapy,[5] chemotherapy,[6] and hormonal and/or biological therapies.[7] The fatigue prevalence is estimated at 25% to 99% while undergoing treatment.[5–8] Henry and colleagues[9] conducted a cross-sectional survey of 1569 patients with cancer. CRF was experienced by 80% of those who received chemotherapy and then radiotherapy. The prevalence of CRF surpasses 75% in patients with metastatic disease.[10–12] Factors such as the population studied, treatment received, and evaluation type (type of screening tool) contribute to the prevalence of fatigue during treatment.[1] However, despite the predominance and negative effect of CRF, this symptom is underreported by patients, and underestimated and undertreated by clinicians.[13] Patients may not talk with their physicians about fatigue because of their fear of not receiving maximum cancer treatment; their belief it is an expected symptom and is untreatable; their belief they will be thought of as a "complainer"; or their belief that fatigue is a sign of recurrent or advancing disease. In response, physicians and other health care providers may not ask about fatigue because they often lack knowledge regarding management and their perception of limited treatment options or because of time constraints in a busy clinical environment. Reports acquired from cancer survivors suggest that fatigue may persevere for a considerable length of time or even years after treatment.[14] Despite some improvement in fatigue symptoms following the first year of treatment completion, approximately 25% to 30% of patients will continue to experience these symptoms up to 5 years after successful completion of treatment and in some cases longer.[15–17] A significant variable driving the assessment and treatment of CRF has been the developing recognition of the negative effect of fatigue on quality of life.[18]

PATHOPHYSIOLOGY

The cause of CRF is often vague. Although unproven, there have been several hypotheses of the pathophysiology of CRF. The hypotheses include serotonin (5-HT) dysregulation, hypothalamic-pituitary-adrenal (HPA) axis dysfunction, circadian rhythm disruption, muscle metabolism/ATP dysregulation, vagal afferent nerve activation, and cytokine dysregulation.

5-HT dysregulation hypothesizes that the malignancy and/or associated treatment causes an expansion in brain 5-HT levels including upregulation of a population of 5-HT receptors resulting in a decreased somatomotor drive, a modified HPA axis function, and a sensation of decreased ability to exhibit physical work.[19]

Another potential cause of fatigue is the aggravation of the HPA axis. This hypothesis suggests that cancer, and/or cancer treatment, modifies the function of the HPA axis, resulting in endocrine changes that cause or add to fatigue.[20]

Circadian rhythms are described as endogenous hereditary and physiologically based patterns that are controlled by the body's "clock." These rhythms operate on a 24-hour cycle and are sensitive to environmental (eg, alterations in light and dark) and psychological factors (eg, stress, anxiety, and illness). Relative to patients with cancer, a few alterations in circadian function have been demonstrated and entail changes in endocrine rhythms (eg, cortisol, melatonin, and prolactin secretion), metabolic processes (eg, temperature and circulating protein levels), the immune system (eg, levels of circulating leukocytes and neutrophils), and rest-activity patterns. Patients with advanced cancer tend to show the greatest rhythm alterations.[21]

Cancer and/or its treatment result in a defect in the pathway for regenerating ATP in skeletal muscle, altering the ability to do mechanical tasks. Patients perceive CRF as feelings of "weakness" and "lack of energy." These feelings may correlate to peripheral fatigue (ie, the muscles have a reduced capacity for contractile response).[19]

The vagal afferent nerve activation hypothesis suggests that cancer as well as its treatment causes a peripheral release of neuroactive agents that initiate vagal afferent nerves, resulting in downregulation of somatic muscle activity and induction of "sickness behavior."[22–24]

The cytokine dysregulation hypothesis involves tumor necrosis factor-alpha (TNF-α) and interleukin-1beta, types of proinflammatory cytokines involved in several systems. TNF has appeared to be related to modifications in central nervous system neurotransmission and changes in behavior such as lethargy and anorexia. Another cytokine associated with fatigue is interferon-alpha.[25]

SCREENING

Screening and managing CRF in patients undergoing active cancer treatment and those after treatment are similar. Additional steps are taken in both depending on fatigue severity.

Various scales to objectively measure fatigue have been used in both clinical and research settings (**Table 1**). The simplest is a scale from 0 to 10, where 0 indicates having no fatigue and 10 refers to the most severe fatigue endured. Cut points have been derived and are consistent with other scales; patients with no fatigue through mild fatigue (scores 0–3) usually have little hindrance in daily activities and should receive education, counseling, and general strategies for fatigue management.[26] General strategies include self-monitoring of fatigue levels, energy conservation, and distraction. Energy conservation includes managing daily activities by setting priorities and allocating more time and energy for important tasks to prevent burnout and avoiding physical inactivity.[27,28]

Patients with moderate (4–6) to severe fatigue (7–10) usually have difficulty with daily activities. In addition to education, counseling, and general strategies for management of fatigue, patients with moderate to severe fatigue require further methodical evaluation, including a focused history with assessment of treatable factors and a physical examination (**Box 1**).

Table 1	
Measures of fatigue for use in patients with cancer	
Unidimensional Measures	**Multidimensional Measures**
Symptom Distress Scale	Revised Piper Fatigue Scale
Fatigue Symptom Inventory	Cancer Fatigue Scale
Brief Fatigue Inventory	Revised Schwartz Cancer Fatigue Scale
Fatigue Severity Scale	The Multidimensional Fatigue Inventory
	The Multidimensional Fatigue Symptom Inventory

Data from Escalante CP, Wang XS. Cancer-related fatigue. In: Yeung S, Escalante CP, Gagel RF, editors. Medical care of cancer patient. Shelton (CT): People's Medical Publishing House; 2009. p. 53–9.

Box 1
Contributory factors in cancer-related fatigue

Symptom burden

Pain

Anxiety and depression

Stress

Sleep disturbances

Obstructive sleep apnea

Restless leg syndrome

Vasomotor symptoms

Insomnia

Nutritional imbalances

Weight/caloric intake changes

Fluid and electrolyte imbalance

Decreased functional status

Physical activity level

Deconditioning

Medical issues

Anemia from various causes

Cardiac dysfunction

Endocrine dysfunction

Pulmonary dysfunction

Renal dysfunction

Neuromuscular complications

Hepatic dysfunction

Rheumatologic disorders

Medications

Sedating agents

Beta-blockers

Other (drug interactions and other medication side effects)

Cancer treatment effects

Chemotherapy

Radiotherapy

Surgery

Bone marrow transplantation

Biologic response modifiers

Hormonal treatment

Immunotherapy

Data from National Comprehensive Cancer Network. Cancer-Related Fatigue (Version 1.2017). Available at: http://www.nccn.org/professionals/physician_gls/pdf/fatigue.pdf. Accessed January 23, 2017.

PATIENT HISTORY, PHYSICAL EXAMINATION, AND DIAGNOSTIC WORKUP

The primary goal in assessing patients presenting with CRF is to acquire a complete and detailed history. The patient history is particularly useful in differentiating between various causes that may be contributing to fatigue. According to the NCCN CRF guidelines, an in-depth fatigue history focusing on onset, patterns, duration, change over time, associated or alleviating factors, interference with function, caregiver availability, activity level, and economic status are key when evaluating a patient with fatigue.[29] Comorbid conditions such as existing coronary disease, hypothyroidism, renal disease, hepatic disease, pulmonary disease, and anemia are imperative to obtain when acquiring patient history because these conditions may contribute to CRF.[29]

The cancer diagnosis, associated treatments, and current cancer status are important factors of the patient history. The relationship of fatigue to cancer recurrence in patients who are thought to be free of disease versus progression in patients with continued disease is an important component driving patients to seek further assessment. Cancer treatments may include chemotherapy, surgery, bone marrow transplantation, immunotherapy, or hormonal treatment. The past medical history may reveal comorbidities that may not be optimally managed and contributing to fatigue. Thorough evaluation of medications is another essential aspect of the patient's history. The medication review should include recent medication changes and use of prescription and over-the-counter medications, supplements, vitamins, and herbal treatments. The social history should be documented, because the use of alcohol or illicit drugs may contribute to fatigue. A detailed review of systems is essential to assess treatable contributing symptoms and should entail questions regarding anemia, pain, depression, anxiety, sleep disturbances, nutritional imbalance, and decreased functional status.[29]

The physical examination is important in identifying key features that may aid in the diagnosis of CRF, especially in the presence of other symptoms. A systematic and meticulous examination of the patient is warranted. Findings such as scleral icterus, pulmonary rales, or a heart murmur may lead to identification of associated symptoms and diagnosis of other medical issues that may be contribute to CRF.

Laboratory evaluation should be done to eliminate other treatable causes of fatigue. The workup should include complete blood cell count with differential, comprehensive metabolic panel to evaluate electrolytes, hepatic and renal functions, and an endocrine panel to evaluate the thyroid function.[29] In men, a testosterone level test should be considered. Further testing is dependent upon findings of the physical examination.

TREATMENT INTERVENTIONS

Based on the patient-specific assessment, reversible key contributory factors for CRF are initially addressed; these treatable factors may include unrelieved pain, emotional distress, sleep disturbance, anemia, metabolic/nutritional/hormonal issues, uncontrolled comorbidities, medication side effects, decreased activity level, and deconditioning.[30] Other specific interventions are grouped into nonpharmacologic and pharmacologic interventions.

Nonpharmacologic Interventions

Nonpharmacologic interventions include psychosocial interventions, exercise, yoga, physically based therapy, dietary management, and sleep therapy. Although more extensive and diverse research is necessary to further validate the significance of interventions for treating CRF, psychosocial interventions and exercise have the most supportive evidence of the nonpharmacologic interventions during active treatment and after treatment.[31,32]

Psychosocial Interventions

Psychosocial interventions include cognitive behavioral therapy (CBT), psychoeducational therapy, and supportive expressive therapy. CBT and psychoeducational therapy have reduced CRF levels and have the strongest evidence (category 1) supporting their use. The efficacy of CBT and psychoeducational therapy in reducing fatigue was demonstrated in different types of studies, including clinical trials, meta-analyses, and other systematic reviews.[33–38]

CBT benefits cancer survivors by promoting behavioral changes that lead to self-care management. Relaxation strategies, such as listening to guided-imagery tapes and taking short naps, are part of self-care management. These therapies are designed to promote expressing emotion and seeking support from others.

Exercise

Physical activity or exercise is another category with the most supportive evidence in reducing CRF (category 1). In a *Cochrane Review* in 2012, 56 randomized controlled trials were identified to examine the effects of exercise in adults with CRF. The experimental group of 1461 participants received exercise interventions and was compared with the control group of 1187; exercise was shown to be statistically more effective than the control group.[39]

Despite sounding counterintuitive, exercise is strongly recommended to all cancer survivors as long as they are not at higher risk of injury (survivors with neuropathy, cardiomyopathy, or other long-term effects of therapy).[29] According to the American Society of Clinical Oncology CRF guidelines, cancer survivors are suggested to participate in 150 minutes of moderate aerobic exercise and 2 to 3 strength-training sessions every week.[1] An individualized exercise program is required with consideration of the cancer survivor's overall medical history, including their current status. Other factors that should be reviewed in planning an exercise regimen include the patient's age and gender, the type of cancer present, the treatment received and currently undergoing, the present physical fitness level and past involvement in physical activities, and the presence of comorbidities and their status. Survivors with significant comorbidities may especially need a thorough medical evaluation before assigning an exercise intervention. Walking programs are a common exercise intervention recommended to most cancer survivors.[40] Other examples of physical exercise training programs found in various studies were stationary cycling, stair-climbing machines, strength and resistance training, swimming, and aerobic classes.[32,41] Some studies allowed participants to choose their preferred type of aerobic exercise.

Yoga

Yoga has been studied in patients with cancer undergoing treatment (chemotherapy, radiotherapy) using randomized controlled trials with improvement of CRF.[42–48] It does have supportive evidence of its effectiveness and is rated category 1. However, additional data are needed in select cancers and in men.

Physically Based Therapy

Acupuncture and massage therapy, the 2 main types of physically based therapy, have been studied for treatment of CRF. Small-sample studies reported that acupuncture and massage had positive effects on alleviating fatigue levels in cancer survivors.[49–51] However, further randomized controlled trials are essential to validate their longer-term effectiveness.

Dietary Management

Cancer and its treatment may disrupt nutritional balances. Many cancer survivors suffer from nutritional issues.[52] Because fatigue symptoms may be improved by proper dietary management, nutritional assessment should be performed for cancer survivors to evaluate changes in weight and caloric intake and imbalances in fluid and electrolytes. Appropriate education focused on a healthy well-balanced diet is essential for all cancer survivors. For those survivors with special nutritional requirements (gastric resection, poor colonic absorption), referral to a dietary specialist may be essential in maintaining nutritional balance.

Sleep Therapy

Sleep disturbances are challenging for cancer survivors because they often exacerbate CRF. Contributory factors to sleep disturbances are frequently anxiety, depression, and daytime napping as well as medication side effects, nutritional characteristics, and nocturnal awakenings. CBT is recommended for sleep improvement; it includes stimulus control, sleep restriction, and sleep hygiene. Examples of stimulus control include setting a consistent sleep schedule going to bed and waking and staying away from caffeine and stimulating activity before bedtime. Sleep restriction includes avoiding long or late daytime naps and limiting time in bed to sleep normally required. Education and counseling on sleep hygiene may be helpful. Symptoms of other sleep-related reversible conditions such as obstructive sleep apnea may be detected during the history-taking and may need further assessment.

Pharmacologic Interventions

The most studied pharmacologic interventions for treating CRF include psychostimulants, antidepressants, corticosteroids, and other complementary agents.

Psychostimulants

Despite weak supporting evidence on the efficacy of psychostimulants, they have been the most frequently prescribed agents in attempting to reduce CRF in cancer survivors. Studies using psychostimulants for treating CRF are often poorly designed with relatively small numbers of participants.

The most common psychostimulants selected for treating CRF are methylphenidate and modafinil. Methylphenidate is a central nervous system stimulant that is approved by the US Food and Drug Administration (FDA) for the treatment of attention-deficit/hyperactivity disorder and narcolepsy[53] (**Table 2**). It is a controlled substance and available in both short-acting and long-acting preparations. The common starting dose for the short-acting preparation of methylphenidate for treating CRF is 5 mg taken orally in the morning and another 5 mg at noon. It has a short plasma half-life of 2 hours with a duration of action lasting 3 to 6 hours with a rapid onset.[54] An advantage of a short-acting dose is flexibility in dose adjustment depending on the level of fatigue at the time of administration; a patient can choose to take a higher dose of methylphenidate when higher levels of fatigue are anticipated. The starting dose for the long-acting preparation is usually 18 mg and is taken orally in the morning. Its duration of action is approximately 12 hours. Individuals uncomfortable with a twice-daily schedule may prefer the long-acting preparation. A meta-analysis on the efficacy in reducing CRF includes 7 randomized

Table 2
Commonly used psychostimulants for treatment of cancer-related fatigue

	Methylphenidate (Ritalin)	Methylphenidate (Concerta)	Modafinil (Provigil)
FDA-approved uses	ADHD Narcolepsy	ADHD	Narcolepsy OSA SWD
Preparation	Short-acting	Long-acting	Short-acting
Starting dose	5 mg orally morning & noon	18 mg orally morning	100 mg orally morning & noon
Maximum dose	1 mg/kg per day	54 mg per day	400 mg orally

Abbreviations: ADHD, attention-deficit/hyperactivity disorder; OSA, obstructive sleep apnea; SWD, shift work disorder.
Data from Escalante CP, Manzullo EF. Fatigue. In: Foxhall LE, Rodriguez MA, editors. Advances in Cancer Survivorship Management. New York: Springer; 2015. p. 361–73.

controlled trials from 2006 to 2014.[55] It demonstrated a superior result in the methylphenidate arm compared with the placebo arm. In this analysis, 661 patients received methylphenidate or a placebo at a minimum of 5 mg daily to a maximum of 36 mg daily (a dosing schedule of 5 mg every 2 hours was allowed for one of the studies).[56–59] However, methylphenidate showed no improvement in fatigue levels in patients with end-stage cancer.[60]

Modafinil is a nonamphetamine central nervous system stimulant that is approved by the FDA for the treatment of narcolepsy, obstructive sleep apnea/hypopnea syndrome, and shift work sleep disorder.[61] Usually, the starting dose of modafinil for treating CRF is 100 mg taken orally in the morning and 100 mg at noon (see **Table 2**). Compared with the findings from the methylphenidate studies, the efficacy of modafinil on CRF showed weaker correlations. A meta-analysis of 3 studies investigating modafinil from 2010 to 2014 reported no statistically significant improvement in fatigue with modafinil treatment.[55] In this meta-analysis, 921 patients received modafinil at a minimum dose of 100 mg daily to a maximum of 200 mg daily or a placebo.

Antidepressants

Antidepressants may benefit patients with cancer when CRF is accompanied by depression.[62–64] They should not be used as a primary treatment of CRF. Placebo-controlled studies of patients with cancer during active treatment showed that antidepressants such as paroxetine and sertraline had no improvement in CRF levels.[62,65–67] However, paroxetine was found to alleviate CRF levels in depressed survivors or when fatigue presented as a symptom of depression.[62–64]

Other Agents

Studies involving corticosteroids for CRF are usually limited to advanced patients with cancer in a palliative care setting due to longer-term toxicity. In these studies, corticosteroids have shown effectiveness in reducing CRF.[68,69] In a multicenter, prospective, observational study, 179 participants with metastatic or locally advanced cancer were treated with corticosteroids (betamethasone, dexamethasone, and prednisolone), and 86 showed a 2-point reduction or more in their fatigue intensity scores.[69]

Limited studies have been done using vitamins and dietary supplements such as coenzyme Q and L-carnitine. Vitamins and supplements have shown no benefit in the treatment of CRF.

Complementary Agents

Ginseng and guarana have been studied for treatment of CRF.[70–74] The data are inconclusive and do not support treatment of CRF. In addition, ginseng does interact with numerous classes of medications, including warfarin, calcium channel blockers, and antiplatelet and thrombolytic agents, and should be carefully monitored for drug interactions if used.

SUMMARY

- CRF is a distressing, persistent, subjective sense of physical, emotional, and/or cognitive tiredness or exhaustion related to cancer or cancer treatment that is not proportional to recent activity and that significantly interferes with usual functioning.[2]
- Screening should be performed at the time of the cancer diagnosis, throughout cancer treatment, and following completion of the essential cancer treatment.
- A fatigue scoring scale (mild-severe) can be used to evaluate fatigue in cancer survivors.
- The general approach to CRF management includes education, counseling, and other strategies. This approach should be used for survivors at all fatigue levels. Cancer survivors with moderate to severe CRF require an additional detailed evaluation.
- Nonpharmacologic interventions include psychosocial interventions, exercise, yoga, physically based therapy, dietary management, and sleep therapy. CBT, psychoeducational therapy, yoga, and exercise have the most supporting evidence for CRF management (category 1).
- The psychostimulant, methylphenidate, is a pharmacologic intervention that may be considered in CRF. It does not have category 1 supporting evidence and is not FDA approved for CRF. Antidepressants may also benefit cancer survivors when CRF and depression are both present. Corticosteroids are usually limited to patients with cancer with advanced disease.

REFERENCES

1. Bower JE. Cancer-related fatigue–mechanisms, risk factors, and treatments. Nat Rev Clin Oncol 2014;11(10):597–609.
2. Mock V, Atkinson A, Barsevick A, et al. NCCN practice guidelines for cancer-related fatigue. Oncology (Williston Park) 2000;14(11a):151–61.
3. Clark EJ, Stovall EL, Leigh S, et al. Imperatives for quality cancer care: access, advocacy, action, and accountability. Silver Spring (MD): National Coalition of Cancer Survivorship; 1996. p. 7–8.
4. de Jong N, Candel MJ, Schouten HC, et al. Prevalence and course of fatigue in breast cancer patients receiving adjuvant chemotherapy. Ann Oncol 2004;15(6): 896–905.
5. Hickok JT, Roscoe JA, Morrow GR, et al. Frequency, severity, clinical course, and correlates of fatigue in 372 patients during 5 weeks of radiotherapy for cancer. Cancer 2005;104(8):1772–8.

6. Jacobsen PB, Hann DM, Azzarello LM, et al. Fatigue in women receiving adjuvant chemotherapy for breast cancer: characteristics, course, and correlates. J Pain Symptom Manage 1999;18(4):233–42.

7. Phillips KM, Pinilla-Ibarz J, Sotomayor E, et al. Quality of life outcomes in patients with chronic myeloid leukemia treated with tyrosine kinase inhibitors: a controlled comparison. Support Care Cancer 2013;21(4):1097–103.

8. Servaes P, Verhagen S, Bleijenberg G. Determinants of chronic fatigue in disease-free breast cancer patients: a cross-sectional study. Ann Oncol 2002; 13(4):589–98.

9. Henry DH, Viswanathan HN, Elkin EP, et al. Symptoms and treatment burden associated with cancer treatment: results from a cross-sectional national survey in the U.S. Support Care Cancer 2008;16(7):791–801.

10. Portenoy RK, Kornblith AB, Wong G, et al. Pain in ovarian cancer patients. Prevalence, characteristics, and associated symptoms. Cancer 1994;74(3):907–15.

11. Ventafridda V, De Conno F, Ripamonti C, et al. Quality-of-life assessment during a palliative care programme. Ann Oncol 1990;1(6):415–20.

12. Curtis EB, Krech R, Walsh TD. Common symptoms in patients with advanced cancer. J Palliat Care 1991;7(2):25–9.

13. Berger AM, Gerber LH, Mayer DK. Cancer-related fatigue: implications for breast cancer survivors. Cancer 2012;118(8 Suppl):2261–9.

14. Haghighat S, Akbari ME, Holakouei K, et al. Factors predicting fatigue in breast cancer patients. Support Care Cancer 2003;11(8):533–8.

15. Bower JE, Ganz PA, Desmond KA, et al. Fatigue in breast cancer survivors: occurrence, correlates, and impact on quality of life. J Clin Oncol 2000;18(4): 743–53.

16. Minton O, Stone P. How common is fatigue in disease-free breast cancer survivors? A systematic review of the literature. Breast Cancer Res Treat 2008; 112(1):5–13.

17. Bower JE, Ganz PA, Desmond KA, et al. Fatigue in long-term breast carcinoma survivors: a longitudinal investigation. Cancer 2006;106(4):751–8.

18. Sobrero A, Puglisi F, Guglielmi A, et al. Fatigue: a main component of anemia symptomatology. Semin Oncol 2001;28(2 Suppl 8):15–8.

19. Andrews P, Morrow GR, Hickok J, et al. Mechanisms and models of fatigue associated with cancer and its treatment: evidence from preclinical and clinical studies. In: Armes J, Krishnasamy M, Higgenson I, editors. Fatigue in Cancer. Oxford: Oxford University Press; 2004. p. 51–87.

20. Cleare AJ. The neuroendocrinology of chronic fatigue syndrome. Endocr Rev 2003;24(2):236–52.

21. Bower JE, Ganz PA, Dickerson SS, et al. Diurnal cortisol rhythm and fatigue in breast cancer survivors. Psychoneuroendocrinology 2005;30(1):92–100.

22. Blackshaw LA, Grundy D. Effects of 5-hydroxytryptamine on discharge of vagal mucosal afferent fibres from the upper gastrointestinal tract of the ferret. J Auton Nerv Syst 1993;45(1):41–50.

23. Ek M, Kurosawa M, Lundeberg T, et al. Activation of vagal afferents after intravenous injection of interleukin-1beta: role of endogenous prostaglandins. J Neurosci 1998;18(22):9471–9.

24. Wang XS. Pathophysiology of cancer-related fatigue. Clin J Oncol Nurs 2008;12(5 Suppl):11–20.

25. Collado-Hidalgo A, Bower JE, Ganz PA, et al. Inflammatory biomarkers for persistent fatigue in breast cancer survivors. Clin Cancer Res 2006;12(9):2759–66.

26. Mendoza TR, Wang XS, Cleeland CS, et al. The rapid assessment of fatigue severity in cancer patients: use of the Brief Fatigue Inventory. Cancer 1999; 85(5):1186–96.

27. Barsevick AM, Dudley W, Beck S, et al. A randomized clinical trial of energy conservation for patients with cancer-related fatigue. Cancer 2004;100(6):1302–10.

28. Richardson A, Ream EK. Self-care behaviours initiated by chemotherapy patients in response to fatigue. Int J Nurs Stud 1997;34(1):35–43.

29. Berger AM, Abernethy AP, Atkinson A, et al. NCCN clinical practice guidelines cancer-related fatigue. J Natl Compr Cancer Netw 2010;8(8):904–31.

30. National Comprehensive Cancer Network. Cancer-Related Fatigue (Version 1.2017). Available at: http://www.nccn.org/professionals/physician_gls/pdf/fatigue.pdf. Accessed January 23, 2017.

31. Mustian KM, Morrow GR, Carroll JK, et al. Integrative nonpharmacologic behavioral interventions for the management of cancer-related fatigue. Oncologist 2007;12(Suppl 1):52–67.

32. Dimeo F, Schwartz S, Wesel N, et al. Effects of an endurance and resistance exercise program on persistent cancer-related fatigue after treatment. Ann Oncol 2008;19(8):1495–9.

33. Duijts SF, Faber MM, Oldenburg HS, et al. Effectiveness of behavioral techniques and physical exercise on psychosocial functioning and health-related quality of life in breast cancer patients and survivors–a meta-analysis. Psychooncology 2011;20(2):115–26.

34. van der Lee ML, Garssen B. Mindfulness-based cognitive therapy reduces chronic cancer-related fatigue: a treatment study. Psychooncology 2012;21(3): 264–72.

35. Jacobsen PB, Donovan KA, Vadaparampil ST, et al. Systematic review and meta-analysis of psychological and activity-based interventions for cancer-related fatigue. Health Psychol 2007;26(6):660–7.

36. Goedendorp MM, Gielissen MF, Verhagen CA, et al. Development of fatigue in cancer survivors: a prospective follow-up study from diagnosis into the year after treatment. J Pain Symptom Manage 2013;45(2):213–22.

37. Kwekkeboom KL, Abbott-Anderson K, Cherwin C, et al. Pilot randomized controlled trial of a patient-controlled cognitive-behavioral intervention for the pain, fatigue, and sleep disturbance symptom cluster in cancer. J Pain Symptom Manage 2012;44(6):810–22.

38. Montgomery GH, David D, Kangas M, et al. Randomized controlled trial of a cognitive-behavioral therapy plus hypnosis intervention to control fatigue in patients undergoing radiotherapy for breast cancer. J Clin Oncol 2014;32(6): 557–63.

39. Cramp F, Byron-Daniel J. Exercise for the management of cancer-related fatigue in adults. Cochrane Database Syst Rev 2012;(11):CD006145.

40. Schmitz KH, Courneya KS, Matthews C, et al. American College of Sports Medicine roundtable on exercise guidelines for cancer survivors. Med Sci Sports Exerc 2010;42(7):1409–26.

41. Tian L, Lu HJ, Lin L, et al. Effects of aerobic exercise on cancer-related fatigue: a meta-analysis of randomized controlled trials. Support Care Cancer 2016;24(2): 969–83.

42. Kiecolt-Glaser JK, Bennett JM, Andridge R, et al. Yoga's impact on inflammation, mood, and fatigue in breast cancer survivors: a randomized controlled trial. J Clin Oncol 2014;32(10):1040–9.

43. Sprod LK, Fernandez ID, Janelsins MC, et al. Effects of yoga on cancer-related fatigue and global side-effect burden in older cancer survivors. J Geriatr Oncol 2015;6(1):8–14.

44. Cramer H, Rabsilber S, Lauche R, et al. Yoga and meditation for menopausal symptoms in breast cancer survivors-A randomized controlled trial. Cancer 2015;121(13):2175–84.

45. Bower JE, Garet D, Sternlieb B, et al. Yoga for persistent fatigue in breast cancer survivors: a randomized controlled trial. Cancer 2012;118(15):3766–75.

46. Taso CJ, Lin HS, Lin WL, et al. The effect of yoga exercise on improving depression, anxiety, and fatigue in women with breast cancer: a randomized controlled trial. J Nurs Res 2014;22(3):155–64.

47. Chakrabarty J, Vidyasagar M, Fernandes D, et al. Effectiveness of pranayama on cancer-related fatigue in breast cancer patients undergoing radiation therapy: a randomized controlled trial. Int J Yoga 2015;8(1):47–53.

48. Chandwani KD, Perkins G, Nagendra HR, et al. Randomized, controlled trial of yoga in women with breast cancer undergoing radiotherapy. J Clin Oncol 2014;32(10):1058–65.

49. Balk J, Day R, Rosenzweig M, et al. Pilot, randomized, modified, double-blind, placebo-controlled trial of acupuncture for cancer-related fatigue. J Soc Integr Oncol 2009;7(1):4–11.

50. Vickers AJ, Straus DJ, Fearon B, et al. Acupuncture for postchemotherapy fatigue: a phase II study. J Clin Oncol 2004;22(9):1731–5.

51. Molassiotis A, Sylt P, Diggins H. The management of cancer-related fatigue after chemotherapy with acupuncture and acupressure: a randomised controlled trial. Complement Ther Med 2007;15(4):228–37.

52. Brown JK. A systematic review of the evidence on symptom management of cancer-related anorexia and cachexia. Oncol Nurs Forum 2002;29(3):517–32.

53. Challman TD, Lipsky JJ. Methylphenidate: its pharmacology and uses. Mayo Clin Proc 2000;75(7):711–21.

54. Faraj BA, Israili ZH, Perel JM, et al. Metabolism and disposition of methylphenidate-14C: studies in man and animals. J Pharmacol Exp Ther 1974;191(3):535–47.

55. Qu D, Zhang Z, Yu X, et al. Psychotropic drugs for the management of cancer-related fatigue: a systematic review and meta-analysis. Eur J Cancer Care 2016;25(6):970–9.

56. Richard PO, Fleshner NE, Bhatt JR, et al. Phase II, randomised, double-blind, placebo-controlled trial of methylphenidate for reduction of fatigue levels in patients with prostate cancer receiving LHRH-agonist therapy. BJU Int 2015; 116(5):744–52.

57. Bruera E, Yennurajalingam S, Palmer JL, et al. Methylphenidate and/or a nursing telephone intervention for fatigue in patients with advanced cancer: a randomized, placebo-controlled, phase II trial. J Clin Oncol 2013;31(19):2421–7.

58. Roth AJ, Nelson C, Rosenfeld B, et al. Methylphenidate for fatigue in ambulatory men with prostate cancer. Cancer 2010;116(21):5102–10.

59. Lower EE, Fleishman S, Cooper A, et al. Efficacy of dexmethylphenidate for the treatment of fatigue after cancer chemotherapy: a randomized clinical trial. J Pain Symptom Manage 2009;38(5):650–62.

60. Mitchell GK, Hardy JR, Nikles CJ, et al. The effect of methylphenidate on fatigue in advanced cancer: an aggregated N-of-1 Trial. J Pain Symptom Manage 2015; 50(3):289–96.

61. Estrada A, Kelley AM, Webb CM, et al. Modafinil as a replacement for dextroamphetamine for sustaining alertness in military helicopter pilots. Aviat Space Environ Med 2012;83(6):556–64.
62. Morrow GR, Hickok JT, Roscoe JA, et al. Differential effects of paroxetine on fatigue and depression: a randomized, double-blind trial from the University of Rochester Cancer Center Community Clinical Oncology Program. J Clin Oncol 2003;21(24):4635–41.
63. Breitbart W, Alici Y. Pharmacologic treatment options for cancer-related fatigue: current state of clinical research. Clin J Oncol Nurs 2008;12(5 Suppl):27–36.
64. Palesh OG, Mustian KM, Peppone LJ, et al. Impact of paroxetine on sleep problems in 426 cancer patients receiving chemotherapy: a trial from the University of Rochester Cancer Center Community Clinical Oncology Program. Sleep Med 2012;13(9):1184–90.
65. Stockler MR, O'Connell R, Nowak AK, et al. Effect of sertraline on symptoms and survival in patients with advanced cancer, but without major depression: a placebo-controlled double-blind randomised trial. Lancet Oncol 2007;8(7): 603–12.
66. Roscoe JA, Morrow GR, Hickok JT, et al. Effect of paroxetine hydrochloride (Paxil) on fatigue and depression in breast cancer patients receiving chemotherapy. Breast Cancer Res Treat 2005;89(3):243–9.
67. Capuron L, Gumnick JF, Musselman DL, et al. Neurobehavioral effects of interferon-alpha in cancer patients: phenomenology and paroxetine responsiveness of symptom dimensions. Neuropsychopharmacology 2002;26(5):643–52.
68. Peuckmann V, Elsner F, Krumm N, et al. Pharmacological treatments for fatigue associated with palliative care. Cochrane Database Syst Rev 2010;(11):CD006788.
69. Matsuo N, Morita T, Matsuda Y, et al. Predictors of responses to corticosteroids for cancer-related fatigue in advanced cancer patients: a multicenter, prospective, observational study. J Pain Symptom Manage 2016;52(1):64–72.
70. Finnegan-John J, Molassiotis A, Richardson A, et al. A systematic review of complementary and alternative medicine interventions for the management of cancer-related fatigue. Integr Cancer Ther 2013;12(4):276–90.
71. Barton DL, Liu H, Dakhil SR, et al. Wisconsin Ginseng (Panax quinquefolius) to improve cancer-related fatigue: a randomized, double-blind trial, N07C2. J Natl Cancer Inst 2013;105(16):1230–8.
72. de Oliveira Campos MP, Riechelmann R, Martins LC, et al. Guarana (Paullinia cupana) improves fatigue in breast cancer patients undergoing systemic chemotherapy. J Altern Complement Med 2011;17(6):505–12.
73. Campos MP, Hassan BJ, Riechelmann R, et al. Cancer-related fatigue: a review. Rev Assoc Med Bras (1992) 2011;57(2):211–9.
74. del Giglio AB, Cubero Dde I, Lerner TG, et al. Purified dry extract of Paullinia cupana (guarana) (PC-18) for chemotherapy-related fatigue in patients with solid tumors: an early discontinuation study. J Diet Suppl 2013;10(4):325–34.

Anxiety and Depression in Cancer Survivors

Jean C. Yi, PhD[a], Karen L. Syrjala, PhD[a,b],*

KEYWORDS

- Anxiety • Depression • Distress • Cancer survivors

KEY POINTS

- Many cancer survivors experience cancer-related fear of recurrence, posttraumatic stress symptoms, anxiety, or depression after completing treatment.
- Anxiety and fear are more common than depression.
- Risk factors are beginning to be understood for these issues. Women and girls, adolescents, and young adults and those who receive intensive treatment are more vulnerable.
- Most of what is known is from breast cancer survivors; more research is needed with diverse cancer survivors.
- Evidence supports several interventions to assist cancer survivors in coping with emotional distress, including behavioral and pharmacologic treatments.

INTRODUCTION

Due to improvements in cancer detection and treatment, two-thirds of those diagnosed with an invasive cancer today will live more than 5 years, with a resulting rising population of long-term survivors.[1,2] With the increasing visibility of survivors has come an awareness that mental health concerns are prominent among survivors' unmet needs, not only anxiety and depression but also various aspects of cancer-related distress. Many survivors adjust to cancer and its associated treatments but a subgroup struggles with emotional adjustment in the survivorship period. It is important to address these mood concerns because they can be barriers to engaging in survivorship care in addition to disrupting quality of life and return to usual activities.[3] This article examines anxiety and depressive symptoms as well as other cancer-related sources of

Disclosure Statement: Both authors have no financial disclosures to report.
[a] Biobehavioral Sciences, Fred Hutchinson Cancer Research Center, 1100 Fairview Avenue North, D5-220, Seattle, WA 98109, USA; [b] Department of Psychiatry and Behavioral Sciences, University of Washington School of Medicine, Box 356560, 1959 NE Pacific Street, Seattle, WA 98195, USA
* Corresponding author. Biobehavioral Sciences, Fred Hutchinson Cancer Research Center, 1100 Fairview Avenue North, D5-220, Seattle, WA 98109
E-mail address: ksyrjala@fredhutch.org

Med Clin N Am 101 (2017) 1099–1113
http://dx.doi.org/10.1016/j.mcna.2017.06.005
0025-7125/17/© 2017 Elsevier Inc. All rights reserved.

medical.theclinics.com

distress in adults who may be survivors of childhood cancer, adolescent and young adult (AYA) cancer survivors, and mature adult cancer survivors, with a brief discussion of treatment options in these populations.

SYMPTOMS

After cancer treatment, many survivors report feeling alone or even abandoned after the intensive support provided during their treatment. Survivors often are fearful and hypervigilant to physical sensations, especially prior to regularly scheduled testing for recurrence. These intermittent, preoccupying anxieties are called fear of recurrence (FOR), although they can also extend to include symptoms of posttraumatic stress, with hyperarousal when exposed to reminders of cancer, avoidance of situations that remind them of treatment, or numbing of emotions.

Many survivors experience emotional distress that does not meet the clinical criteria for anxiety disorder or major depression. Because cancer survivors have numerous sources of distress that increase their potential for adjustment reactions, and to reduce the negative stigma of mental health terms, these common reactions are categorized as distress. The National Comprehensive Cancer Network distress guideline describes distress as extending along a continuum, ranging from common feelings of vulnerability, sadness, and fears of recurrence to disabling depression, anxiety, trauma, panic, and existential crisis.[4]

According to psychiatric diagnosis criteria,[5] a generalized anxiety diagnosis requires excessive anxiety or worry that is difficult to control and impairs function, along with at least 3 of the following symptoms most of the time for the past 6 months:

- Restlessness or feeling keyed up or on edge
- Being easily fatigued
- Difficulty concentrating
- Irritability
- Muscle tension
- Sleep disruptions

A major depression diagnosis requires at least 5 of the following symptoms most of the time in the past 2 weeks:

- Sadness; feeling hopeless, empty, or depressed
- Loss of interest or pleasure in most activities
- Significant changes in weight or appetite
- Sleep disruptions, including sleeping too much or too little
- Psychomotor slowing or agitation that is observable by others
- Fatigue or loss of energy
- Feelings of guilt or worthlessness or feeling like a burden
- Difficulty concentrating or indecisiveness
- Thoughts of being better off dead or active suicidal thoughts or plans

DIAGNOSTIC TESTS

Given the scope of mood problems cancer survivors may experience, clinicians need easy-to-administer methods for screening so that they can make appropriate recommendations and referrals. Numerous methods for screening and diagnosing mental health needs in survivors have been validated that balance ease of use and sensitivity and specificity for defining treatment needs. Many of these measures can be administered in print or online versions, although clinical interview is equally useful and allows for more nuanced understanding of a patient's sources of concern, possible medical or pharmacologic factors affecting mood, and potential responses to recommendations. The National Comprehensive Cancer Network has guidelines for screening distress to assist health care professionals.[6] A commonly recommended measure is the distress thermometer (DT), a simple oral or printed measure that asks patients to rate their distress from 0 (no distress) to 10 (extreme distress). The DT can be used as a screening tool to determine need for further screening using a cutpoint of 5. When compared with structured clinical interviews, however, the DT lacks sensitivity and specificity, and the high rate of false positives could render the single item difficult to use in practice.[7] Therefore, the DT should not be used as a stand-alone screening tool, but if a patient scores 4 or higher a further screening may be needed.[8,9] An alternative is the Patient Health Questionnaire (PHQ)-4, designed with the 2 key depression and anxiety items required for diagnosis.[10] For this measure, a cutpoint of 3 or more provides optimal sensitivity and specificity. It is important to recognize, however, that both the DT and PHQ-4 indicate a need for further screening and do not in themselves constitute sufficient evaluation for diagnosis or treatment.

Somewhat longer measures provide more diagnostic details for depression, anxiety, or posttraumatic stress disorder (PTSD).[11] In a randomized trial using the PHQ-9 to screen hematopoietic cell transplant survivors, the survivors with higher scores wanted the measure to be used in future visits.[12] Screening can stimulate discussions between survivors and providers about these concerns. Furthermore, providers report more satisfaction with the management of psychological issues and of the overall visit.[12] **Table 1** is a list of potential screening tools to use, some of which are discussed in this article.

DIFFERENTIAL DIAGNOSIS

Making a differential diagnosis can be critical with cancer survivors because many of the symptoms of anxiety and depression overlap with other problems survivors report, such as cognitive difficulties and fatigue. Because mood symptoms overlap with each other, clinicians need a thoughtful screening plan to allow differential diagnosis that can help determine a specific treatment strategy. It is important to recognize that a survivor may have an agitated depression with symptoms of both anxiety and depression. Similarly, some of the symptoms for posttraumatic stress also indicate depression or anxiety, for example, loss of interest, irritability, restlessness, difficulty

Table 1
Potential screening tools for anxiety and depression

Measure Name	Concept Measured	Number of Items	Cutoff Score
PHQ-9[13]	Depressive symptoms	9	≥ 10
Generalized Anxiety Disorder Screener[14]	Anxiety symptoms	7	>10
HADS[15]	Anxiety and depressive symptoms, total distress score	14	HADS–depression ≥ 5 HADS–anxiety ≥ 7
PTSD checklist for *Diagnostic and Statistical Manual of Mental Disorders* (fifth edition)[16]	PTSSs	20	>33
Impact of Events Scale[17]	PTSSs	22	≥ 24

Data from Refs.[13–17]

concentrating, or insomnia. Therefore, it is important to either used diagnostic tools that allow for distinguishing these syndromes or the ability to refer to qualified mental health specialists after a more broad screening, such as with the DT or PHQ-4.

ANXIETY AND DEPRESSION IN DIFFERENT POPULATIONS OF SURVIVORS

This section reviews the literature on anxiety and depression in adult survivors of childhood cancer, AYAs, and adult survivors. Within each section, prevalence, risk factors, and trajectories for various mood issues are discussed.

Adult Survivors of Childhood Cancer

Survivors of childhood cancers have been most extensively studied by the Childhood Cancer Survivor Study (CCSS), which has tracked more than 20,000 survivors across the United States. Analysis from the CCSS cohort found that 11% of the survivors had both elevated anxiety and depressive symptoms compared with 5% in the sibling controls.[18] Although most survivors did not meet criteria for a diagnosis of PTSD, many survivors did report posttraumatic stress symptoms (PTSSs), which do not meet clinical criteria for a diagnosis of PTSD. PTSSs can be thought of as a subclinical syndrome relative to PTSD, where some of the symptoms of PTSD are present and disrupt quality of life but do not meet clinical criteria. In contrast to CCSS, a cohort of Dutch childhood cancer survivors found no difference in anxiety or depression between the survivors and controls.[19] In the CCSS cohort, those with chronic health conditions, such as cardiovascular, endocrine, or pulmonary issues, also had higher levels of anxiety and PTSSs.[20]

CCSS has examined the longitudinal course of anxiety and depressive symptoms in childhood survivors who are now adults.[21] Although most report few to no mood symptoms, approximately 9% reported persistent depressive symptoms suggesting a clinical diagnosis of depression and approximately 5% reported anxiety symptoms suggesting a clinical diagnosis of anxiety. Another group reported increasing symptoms over time: 10% for depression and approximately 12% for anxiety. Increasing mood symptoms were related to the survivors' perceptions that their health was worsening. This finding underlines the need continuing evaluation of mood in young adult survivors.

Adolescent and Young Adult Cancer Survivors

AYA survivors are increasingly recognized as a group with emotional needs that differ from either childhood cancer survivors or older adults. Although definitions of AYA age range may vary, the most widely used definition is those diagnosed between ages 15 and 39.[22] In a cohort of hematologic malignancy survivors that used semistructured interviews, 23% met criteria for anxiety, 28% met criteria for depression, and 13% met criteria for PTSSs.[23] In a sample of Australian AYAs, almost half were classified as above the cutoff score for PTSSs.[24] FOR is also common in young adult cancer survivors. Just over half of young adult breast cancer survivors in 1 study reported moderate to high levels of FOR.[25] Another study comparing AYA survivors to controls found no differences in anxiety or depressive symptoms but the AYA survivors did report more PTSSs.[26] Other cohorts of AYAs that were much larger (between N = 300 and N = 6000) found that AYAs reported more distress than controls.[27–29] These inconsistent findings may be due to differing populations of survivors, methodologies, or measures used.

In considering risk factors for impaired mood in AYA survivors, women and girls consistently report more depressive symptoms than young women without a history of cancer or than male survivors. This was found in the National Longitudinal Study of Adolescent Health[30] and the Australian cohort study (described previously).[24] The Australian study identified additional risk factors for elevated distress, which included lower social support, low self-image, and identity issues. More intensive treatment also is predictive of more distress.[31] FOR may be maintained in survivors if they are unable to talk about the cancer experience with their partners.[25] This highlights the importance both of opportunities to process the cancer experience and of tracking these symptoms at least annually in AYAs to identify those with a need for treatment before negative moods become chronic.

Adult Cancer Survivors

Anxiety symptoms

Most survivors are diagnosed as mature adults (over age 40). Approximately 18% to 20% of long-term cancer adult survivors report anxiety symptoms.[32–35] Using the Hospital Anxiety and Depression Scale (HADS) with a cohort of survivors 6 monhts and 12 months postdiagnosis, 22% and 21%, respectively, were higher than the cutpoint of 8.[33] Having higher scores at 6 months predicted higher scores at 12 months. Women and girls had twice the relative risk of anxiety than men and boys. Other identified risk factors for anxiety in adult survivors have included shorter time since diagnosis and a higher number of comorbid conditions[36] as well as younger age, living alone, and a diagnosis of lung cancer or melanoma.[35] A prospective, longitudinal study that documented trajectories of mood symptoms over time found 4 different trajectories in breast cancer survivors assessed over a 2-year follow-up: (1) high stable, (2) high decrease, (3) mild decrease, and (4) low decrease.[37] Financial difficulties, lower global health, and lower functional status were predictive of being in the high stable trajectory.

Posttraumatic stress disorder

PTSSs are common in cancer survivors although full PTSD diagnosis is seen less often. Reported rates vary depending on the population studied because risk factors depend on the intensity of treatment and age among other factors. A meta-analysis of PTSD comparing survivors and controls found that survivors were more likely to have PTSD (odds ratio 1.66; 95% CI, 1.09–2.52).[38] In a sample of long-term testicular cancer survivors who were 11 years postdiagnosis, just over 10% had either subclinical or full PTSD.[39] In a sample of hematopoietic cell transplant survivors, 15% met criteria for PTSD over a period from pretransplant to 1 year post-transplant.[40] Survivors who were younger, diagnosed with later-stage disease, and who recently completed cancer treatment were at risk for PTSD.[38] Pain was associated with higher PTSD levels as well as being female.

PTSSs do not meet the level of the clinical diagnosis of PTSD yet can still be troubling for survivors and interfere with functioning. A study of non–Hodgkin lymphoma survivors found that 37% reported PTSSs.[41] Factors associated with PTSSs include the following[41–43]:

- Lower educational attainment
- Single relationship status
- Lower income (<$20,000)
- Unemployment
- Poor social support
- Racial minorities
- More recent diagnosis
- Younger age at diagnosis
- Greater perceived negative impact of cancer
- Intensity of cancer treatment

Fear of recurrence

As discussed previously, FOR is common in cancer survivors. Approximately 80% of respondents to a national survey of cancer survivors reported some level of FOR as a concern.[44] Even for long-term cancer survivors (median 5 years post-treatment), 38% of colorectal cancer survivors reported high levels of FOR.[45] In another large cohort (>10,000 participants), 50% reported FOR.[46] Attentional bias, a tendency to focus on threat-related stimuli, could be a factor that explains FOR in breast cancer survivors.[47] As an example, Custers and colleagues[47] evaluated women who were either high or low in FOR and found that regardless of the level of FOR, these women had longer reaction times to a task that required them to process cancer-threatening words than healthy controls. This study was conducted in a hospital setting so the breast cancer survivors may have been mentally primed for these cancer words. In another study, breast cancer patients were assessed prior to surgery and 6 months postsurgery for risk factors associated with higher FOR.[48] Risk factors for higher FOR scores at 6 months after treatment included, paradoxically, living with someone compared with living alone as well as greater changes in spiritual life, higher-state anxiety, more self-reported difficulty coping, and reported more distress due to family members. The investigators recognized that living with a partner may be counterintuitive to higher levels of FOR, but they did posit that if a person has low coping self-efficacy, this person may have difficulty navigating the relationships in the context of cancer. Other research has defined risk factors as female gender, age less than 60 years, 5 years to 7 years postdiagnosis, social isolation, less than 10 years of education, and survivors who had a recurrence.[49] Women who had the greatest declines in their FOR scores over time were those who had better physical health along with higher FOR scores at the time of enrollment.[48] In breast cancer survivors who were getting their mammograms, women who reported greater perceived risk, lower coping self-efficacy, and greater reassurance-seeking behaviors were more likely to be in the higher FOR group.[50] Unsurprisingly, FOR tends to increase around the time of scans or other testing for recurrence.[51] FOR may be important to address because it has been related with negative health behaviors, such as smoking and lower levels of physical activity.[46]

Distress

The emotional distress many survivors may experience may not reach the level of a clinical disorder, such as depression or anxiety. Preoperative levels of distress as measured by the DT has predicted postoperative pain 4 months and 8 months after breast surgery.[52] Thus, distress may be important to monitor to prevent other symptoms or other behaviors, such as smoking in survivors.[53] The DT is not only a single-item question but also offers respondents the opportunity to mark which aspects of their lives are distressing. Financial concerns, limited mobility, and sleep problems are associated with distress.[54] Other risk factors for elevated distress vary depending on the population studied. The Health Information National Trends Survey study has found that African American survivors report higher levels of distress compared with other survivors and noncancer controls.[55] Gay and bisexual prostate cancer survivors also report more distress than heterosexual prostate cancer survivors.[56] Married prostate cancer survivors with lower levels of partner support and unmarried survivors reported more distress than married survivors with high levels of partner support.[57] Distress can be a long-term problem for cancer survivors; a longitudinal study of colorectal cancer survivors who were 5 years postdiagnosis found that one-third of the sample reported high levels of distress.[58] The study also found that younger men who had late-stage disease, lower educational attainment, and poorer social support were likely to have higher levels of distress over the course of survivorship.

Depressive symptoms

Negative mood symptoms, such as anxiety, FOR, PTSSs, and depression, often co-occur. In a population-based, longitudinal study, 9% of survivors had both anxiety and depressive symptoms.[33] In a sample of colorectal and head and neck cancer survivors, exposure to childhood trauma was associated with higher depressive symptoms.[59] When screening depression alone, the prevalence of these symptoms that are above cutpoints for depression range from 12% to 14%.[33,60–66] A meta-analysis of major depression diagnosed with interviews in the nonpalliative care setting found a prevalence of 16%.[67] This was confirmed in women with breast cancer who were followed 4 months after their diagnosis and over the course of 1 year were assessed a total of 7 times using a clinical interview and questionnaire. In these closely tracked women, 17% met criteria for a major depressive episode.[68]

Physical symptoms can be associated with depressive symptoms.[69] As an example, oral cancer survivors who reported dental health, problems with smelling, and issues with range of motion were associated with both depressive and anxiety symptoms.[70] In prostate cancer survivors, men with higher levels of urinary and androgen deprivation therapy symptoms reported higher levels of depressive symptoms.[64] Reduced sexual function by head and neck cancers also has been associated with depressive symptoms.[66] In a Medicare sample of colorectal cancer survivors, ethnic minorities having 2 or more comorbidities and difficulties in daily living were associated with more depressive symptoms.[71] Lack of receipt of a survivorship care plan, which is mandated by the American College of Surgeons,[72] has also been associated with higher depressive symptoms.[73]

Risk factors for depressive symptoms include

- In a heterogeneous sample of adult cancer survivors, a diagnosis of melanoma, survivors not in remission, and smoking[33]
- Women and girls[61]
- A higher number of comorbid conditions[36,63,74]
- Negative body image for women[75,76]
- Financial problems[64,71,77,78]
- Within the first 2 years of survivorship[79]
- Prior history of depression[33,35]
- A sedentary lifestyle[33,35]
- Loneliness[80]

Longitudinal studies have examined the different trajectories of depressive symptoms following a cancer diagnosis. Breast cancer survivors (N = 653) were assessed 4 times (baseline, 6 months, 12 months, and 18 months) and 6 trajectories were identified.[81] Most of the sample could be classified as having very low or low depressive symptoms whereas 29% had consistently borderline scores. Another 11% had high depressive scores at baseline and declined over time but was still above the cutoff; 7% had increasing depressive symptoms whereas a very small percentage (1%) reported very high scores at all of the timepoints. Stanton and colleagues[68] found similar trajectories in their sample of breast cancer survivors.

TREATMENT OPTIONS

Evidence from randomized controlled trials indicate that several behavioral approaches are effective in improving mood in cancer survivors, although a majority of studies have been done in female breast cancer survivors. Therefore, all these interventions need further testing with diverse groups of survivors, in particular men. Cognitive behavioral therapy is effective in reducing mood symptoms in cancer survivors.[82–84] Mindfulness-based approaches also have demonstrated efficacy in reducing anxiety and depressive symptoms.[85–89] In a small study, hypnosis has reduced anxiety symptoms in breast cancer survivors.[90] Self-management strategies also are effective in decreasing distress.[91–93] Modes of intervention delivery are rapidly changing and the Internet and social networking modalities may be attractive options for psychosocial interventions because many survivors already use these resources for cancer information.[70,92–99] Telehealth approaches may improve access to mental health resources, especially for those with limited online access or lack of online skill.[84,100,101] Physical activity interventions also reduce depressive and anxiety symptoms in breast cancer survivors.[102] In a study of prostate cancer survivors, however, in which depressive symptoms and anxiety were secondary outcomes, there was no effect of the physical activity intervention on mood.[103]

Medications provide additional options for regulating mood. A small study using selective serotonin reuptake inhibitors and serotonin-norepinephrine reuptake inhibitors for the treatment of hot flashes in breast cancer survivors found reductions in depressive symptoms with both types of medications.[104] In a medical chart review of more than 16,000 breast cancer survivors, there was no indication of an increased risk of recurrence when concurrently taking tamoxifen and antidepressants although caution is still recommended for prescribing medications with cytochrome P450 interactions, specifically fluoxetine, paroxetine, sertraline, bupropion, fluvoxamine, and nefazodone.[6,105] Gabapentin has been tested in a 3-arm randomized controlled trial with breast cancer survivors comparing 300 mg, 900 mg, and a placebo, and the 300-mg dose condition had the best outcomes except for those with the highest levels of anxiety.[106] Gabapentin, like venlafaxine, is also effective for hot flashes so these medications could be beneficial in reducing multiple symptoms. With the options available to treat mood symptoms, and the lack of evidence for the superiority of one treatment over another, asking survivors their preferences for treatment can be a way to engage in shared decision making and potentially to improve adherence (see **Table 2** for a summary of evidenced-based interventions in cancer survivors).

Table 2
Evidence-based interventions for cancer survivors

Type of Intervention	Modality	Cancer Populations with Evidence	Outcomes
Cognitive behavioral therapy[82–84]	Face to face, telehealth	Breast, hematopoietic cell transplant	Depressive symptoms, anxiety, posttraumatic stress
Mindfulness-based stress reduction[85–89]	Face to face	Breast	Depressive symptoms, anxiety, FOR
Hypnosis[90]	Face to face	Breast	Depressive symptoms
Self-management[91–93]	Web-based	Breast, mixed cancer sites	Distress
Physical activity[95,102]	Face to face, Web-based	Breast	Depressive symptoms, anxiety
Gabapentin[106]	Face to face	Breast	Anxiety

Data from Refs.[82–93,95,102,106]

SUMMARY

Many survivors cope well with cancer and its associated treatments. For a subgroup of survivors, however, anxiety, depression, fears, and distress can linger for up to 10 years after treatment.[107] For some of the issues discussed in this article, such as FOR, no standardized definitions exist, which makes comparing research results difficult.[108] More research is needed with diverse survivors on many levels: types and stages of cancer, racial/ethnic diversity, sexual minorities, and rural survivors, to name a few groups. Improved screening methods also need to be developed and validated to monitor survivors' symptoms over time and make appropriate referrals. When looking at the various treatment options, it is clear that most interventions have been tested only with breast cancer survivors, and treatments with patients who have other diagnoses need to be tested. Information also is lacking about survivors who were not treated at large cancer centers.[109] In short, cancer survivors have long-term increased risk for mood disruptions and evidence-based treatments exist that can relieve their distress.

REFERENCES

1. American Cancer Society. Cancer treatment & survivorship facts & figures 2016-2017. Atlanta (GA): American Cancer Society; 2016.
2. Miller KD, Siegel RL, Lin CC, et al. Cancer treatment and survivorship statistics, 2016. CA Cancer J Clin 2016;66(4):271–89.
3. Berg CJ, Stratton E, Esiashvili N, et al. Young adult cancer survivors' experience with cancer treatment and follow-up care and perceptions of barriers to engaging in recommended care. J Cancer Educ 2016;31(3):430–42.
4. Holland JC, Andersen B, Breitbart WS, et al. Distress management. J Natl Compr Canc Netw 2013;11(2):190–209.
5. Vahia VN. Diagnostic and Statistical Manual of Mental Disorders. 5th edition. Arlington (VA): American Psychiatric Association; 2013.
6. Denlinger CS, Ligibel JA, Are M, et al. NCCN guidelines insights: survivorship, version 1.2016. J Natl Compr Cancer Netw 2016;14(6):715–24.
7. Jacobsen PB. Screening for psychological distress in cancer patients: challenges and opportunities. J Clin Oncol 2007;25(29):4526–7.
8. Recklitis CJ, Blackmon JE, Chang G. Screening young adult cancer survivors for distress with the distress thermometer: comparisons with a structured clinical diagnostic interview. Cancer 2016;122(2):296–303.
9. Mitchell AJ. Pooled results from 38 analyses of the accuracy of distress thermometer and other ultra-short methods of detecting cancer-related mood disorders. J Clin Oncol 2007;25(29):4670–81.
10. Kroenke K, Spitzer RL, Williams JB, et al. An ultra-brief screening scale for anxiety and depression: the PHQ-4. Psychosomatics 2009;50(6):613–21.
11. Costa DS, Smith AB, Fardell JE. The sum of all fears: conceptual challenges with measuring fear of cancer recurrence. Support Care Cancer 2016;24(1):1–3.
12. Hoodin F, Zhao L, Carey J, et al. Impact of psychological screening on routine outpatient care of hematopoietic cell transplantation survivors. Biol Blood Marrow Transplant 2013;19(10):1493–7.
13. Kroenke K, Spitzer RL, Williams JB, et al. The patient health questionnaire somatic, anxiety, and depressive symptom scales: a systematic review. Gen Hosp Psychiatry 2010;32(4):345–59.
14. Spitzer RL, Kroenke K, Williams JB, et al. A brief measure for assessing generalized anxiety disorder: the GAD-7. Arch Intern Med 2006;166(10):1092–7.

15. Mitchell AJ, Meader N, Symonds P. Diagnostic validity of the hospital anxiety and depression scale (HADS) in cancer and palliative settings: a meta-analysis. J Affect Disord 2010;126(3):335–48.

16. Blevins CA, Weathers FW, Davis MT, et al. The posttraumatic stress disorder checklist for DSM-5 (PCL-5): development and initial psychometric evaluation. J Trauma Stress 2015;28(6):489–98.

17. Weiss DS, Marmar CR. The impact of event scale - revised. In: Wilson J, Keane TM, editors. Assessing psychological trauma and PTSD. New York: Guilford; 1996. p. 399–411.

18. D'Agostino NM, Edelstein K, Zhang N, et al. Comorbid symptoms of emotional distress in adult survivors of childhood cancer. Cancer 2016;122(20):3215–24.

19. van der Geest IM, van Dorp W, Hop WC, et al. Emotional distress in 652 Dutch very long-term survivors of childhood cancer, using the hospital anxiety and depression scale (HADS). J Pediatr Hematol Oncol 2013;35(7):525–9.

20. Vuotto SC, Krull KR, Li C, et al. Impact of chronic disease on emotional distress in adult survivors of childhood cancer: A report from the Childhood Cancer Survivor Study. Cancer 2017;123(3):521–8.

21. Brinkman TM, Zhu L, Zeltzer LK, et al. Longitudinal patterns of psychological distress in adult survivors of childhood cancer. Br J Cancer 2013;109(5): 1373–81.

22. National Cancer Institute. Available at: https://www.cancer.gov/types/aya. Accessed April 3, 2017.

23. Muffly LS, Hlubocky FJ, Khan N, et al. Psychological morbidities in adolescent and young adult blood cancer patients during curative-intent therapy and early survivorship. Cancer 2016;122(6):954–61.

24. McCarthy MC, McNeil R, Drew S, et al. Psychological distress and posttraumatic stress symptoms in adolescents and young adults with cancer and their parents. J Adolesc Young Adult Oncol 2016;5(4):322–9.

25. Cohee AA, Adams RN, Johns SA, et al. Long-term fear of recurrence in young breast cancer survivors and partners. Psychooncology 2017;26(1):22–8.

26. Kamibeppu K, Sato I, Honda M, et al. Mental health among young adult survivors of childhood cancer and their siblings including posttraumatic growth. J Cancer Surviv 2010;4(4):303–12.

27. Kaul S, Avila JC, Mutambudzi M, et al. Mental distress and health care use among survivors of adolescent and young adult cancer: a cross-sectional analysis of the National Health Interview Survey. Cancer 2017;123(5):869–78.

28. Prasad PK, Hardy KK, Zhang N, et al. Psychosocial and neurocognitive outcomes in adult survivors of adolescent and early young adult cancer: a report from the childhood cancer survivor study. J Clin Oncol 2015;33(23):2545–52.

29. Salsman JM, Garcia SF, Yanez B, et al. Physical, emotional, and social health differences between posttreatment young adults with cancer and matched healthy controls. Cancer 2014;120(15):2247–54.

30. Cantrell MA, Posner MA. Psychological distress between young adult female survivors of childhood cancer and matched female cohorts surveyed in the adolescent health study. Cancer Nurs 2014;37(4):271–7.

31. Kazak AE, Derosa BW, Schwartz LA, et al. Psychological outcomes and health beliefs in adolescent and young adult survivors of childhood cancer and controls. J Clin Oncol 2010;28(12):2002–7.

32. Mitchell AJ, Ferguson DW, Gill J, et al. Depression and anxiety in long-term cancer survivors compared with spouses and healthy controls: a systematic review and meta-analysis [review]. Lancet Oncol 2013;14(8):721–32.

33. Boyes AW, Girgis A, D'Este CA, et al. Prevalence and predictors of the short-term trajectory of anxiety and depression in the first year after a cancer diagnosis: a population-based longitudinal study. J Clin Oncol 2013;31(21):2724–9.

34. Jarrett N, Scott I, Addington-Hall J, et al. Informing future research priorities into the psychological and social problems faced by cancer survivors: a rapid review and synthesis of the literature. Eur J Oncol Nurs 2013;17(5):510–20.

35. Boyes AW, Girgis A, D'Este C, et al. Flourishing or floundering? Prevalence and correlates of anxiety and depression among a population-based sample of adult cancer survivors 6months after diagnosis. J Affect Disord 2011;135(1–3): 184–92.

36. Braamse AM, van Turenhout ST, Terhaar Sive Droste JS, et al. Factors associated with anxiety and depressive symptoms in colorectal cancer survivors. Eur J Gastroenterol Hepatol 2016;28(7):831–5.

37. Saboonchi F, Petersson LM, Wennman-Larsen A, et al. Trajectories of anxiety among women with breast cancer: a proxy for adjustment from acute to transitional survivorship. J Psychosoc Oncol 2015;33(6):603–19.

38. Swartzman S, Booth JN, Munro A, et al. Posttraumatic stress disorder after cancer diagnosis in adults: a meta-analysis. Depress Anxiety 2017;34(4):327–39.

39. Dahl AA, Ostby-Deglum M, Oldenburg J, et al. Aspects of posttraumatic stress disorder in long-term testicular cancer survivors: cross-sectional and longitudinal findings. J Cancer Surviv 2016;10(5):842–9.

40. Esser P, Kuba K, Scherwath A, et al. Posttraumatic stress disorder symptomatology in the course of allogeneic HSCT: a prospective study. J Cancer Surviv 2017;11(2):203–10.

41. Smith SK, Zimmerman S, Williams CS, et al. Post-traumatic stress outcomes in non-Hodgkin's lymphoma survivors. J Clin Oncol 2008;26(6):934–41.

42. Stuber ML, Meeske KA, Krull KR, et al. Prevalence and predictors of posttraumatic stress disorder in adult survivors of childhood cancer. Pediatrics 2010; 125(5):e1124–34.

43. Smith SK, Zimmerman S, Williams CS, et al. Post-traumatic stress symptoms in long-term non-Hodgkin's lymphoma survivors: does time heal? J Clin Oncol 2011;29(34):4526–33.

44. Beckjord EB, Reynolds KA, van Londen GJ, et al. Population-level trends in posttreatment cancer survivors' concerns and associated receipt of care: results from the 2006 and 2010 LIVESTRONG surveys. J Psychosoc Oncol 2014;32(2):125–51.

45. Custers JA, Gielissen MF, Janssen SH, et al. Fear of cancer recurrence in colorectal cancer survivors. Support Care Cancer 2016;24(2):555–62.

46. Fisher A, Beeken RJ, Heinrich M, et al. Health behaviours and fear of cancer recurrence in 10 969 colorectal cancer (CRC) patients. Psychooncology 2016; 25(12):1434–40.

47. Custers JA, Becker ES, Gielissen MF, et al. Selective attention and fear of cancer recurrence in breast cancer survivors. Ann Behav Med 2015;49(1):66–73.

48. Dunn LB, Langford DJ, Paul SM, et al. Trajectories of fear of recurrence in women with breast cancer. Support Care Cancer 2015;23(7):2033–43.

49. Koch-Gallenkamp L, Bertram H, Eberle A, et al. Fear of recurrence in long-term cancer survivors-do cancer type, sex, time since diagnosis, and social support matter? Health Psychol 2016;35(12):1329–33.

50. McGinty HL, Small BJ, Laronga C, et al. Predictors and patterns of fear of cancer recurrence in breast cancer survivors. Health Psychol 2016;35(1):1–9.

51. Ozga M, Aghajanian C, Myers-Virtue S, et al. A systematic review of ovarian cancer and fear of recurrence. Palliat Support Care 2015;13(6):1771–80.

52. Mejdahl MK, Mertz BG, Bidstrup PE, et al. Preoperative distress predicts persistent pain after breast cancer treatment: a prospective cohort study. J Natl Compr Cancer Netw 2015;13(8):995–1003 [quiz: 1003].

53. Poghosyan H, Darwish SA, Kim SS, et al. The association between social support and smoking status in cancer survivors with frequent and infrequent mental distress: results from 10 US states, 2010. J Cancer Surviv 2016;10(6):1078–88.

54. VanHoose L, Black LL, Doty K, et al. An analysis of the distress thermometer problem list and distress in patients with cancer. Support Care Cancer 2015; 23(5):1225–32.

55. Apenteng BA, Hansen AR, Opoku ST, et al. Racial disparities in emotional distress among cancer survivors: insights from the Health Information National Trends Survey (HINTS). J Cancer Educ 2016. [Epub ahead of print].

56. Ussher JM, Perz J, Kellett A, et al. Health-related quality of life, psychological distress, and sexual changes following prostate cancer: a comparison of gay and bisexual men with heterosexual men. J Sex Med 2016;13(3):425–34.

57. Kamen C, Mustian KM, Heckler C, et al. The association between partner support and psychological distress among prostate cancer survivors in a nationwide study. J Cancer Surviv 2015;9(3):492–9.

58. Dunn J, Ng SK, Holland J, et al. Trajectories of psychological distress after colorectal cancer. Psychooncology 2013;22(8):1759–65.

59. Archer JA, Hutchison IL, Dorudi S, et al. Interrelationship of depression, stress and inflammation in cancer patients: a preliminary study. J Affect Disord 2012;143(1–3):39–46.

60. Chen AM, Daly ME, Vazquez E, et al. Depression among long-term survivors of head and neck cancer treated with radiation therapy. JAMA Otolaryngol Head Neck Surg 2013;139(9):885–9.

61. Jim HS, Sutton SK, Jacobsen PB, et al. Risk factors for depression and fatigue among survivors of hematopoietic cell transplantation. Cancer 2016;122(8): 1290–7.

62. Mosher CE, Winger JG, Given BA, et al. Mental health outcomes during colorectal cancer survivorship: a review of the literature. Psychooncology 2016; 25(11):1261–70.

63. Rottmann N, Hansen DG, Hagedoorn M, et al. Depressive symptom trajectories in women affected by breast cancer and their male partners: a nationwide prospective cohort study. J Cancer Surviv 2016;10(5):915–26.

64. Sharp L, O'Leary E, Kinnear H, et al. Cancer-related symptoms predict psychological wellbeing among prostate cancer survivors: results from the PiCTure study. Psychooncology 2016;25(3):282–91.

65. Smith AB, Butow P, Olver I, et al. The prevalence, severity, and correlates of psychological distress and impaired health-related quality of life following treatment for testicular cancer: a survivorship study. J Cancer Surviv 2016;10(2):223–33.

66. Suzuki M, Deno M, Myers M, et al. Anxiety and depression in patients after surgery for head and neck cancer in Japan. Palliat Support Care 2016;14(3): 269–77.

67. Mitchell AJ, Chan M, Bhatti H, et al. Prevalence of depression, anxiety, and adjustment disorder in oncological, haematological, and palliative-care settings: a meta-analysis of 94 interview-based studies. Lancet Oncol 2011;12(2): 160–74.

68. Stanton AL, Wiley JF, Krull JL, et al. Depressive episodes, symptoms, and trajectories in women recently diagnosed with breast cancer. Breast Cancer Res Treat 2015;154(1):105–15.

69. Vehling S, Mehnert A, Hartmann M, et al. Anxiety and depression in long-term testicular germ cell tumor survivors. Gen Hosp Psychiatry 2016;38:21–5.

70. Badr H, Lipnick D, Gupta V, et al. Survivorship challenges and information needs after radiotherapy for oral cancer. J Cancer Educ 2016. [Epub ahead of print].

71. Clark CJ, Fino NF, Liang JH, et al. Depressive symptoms in older long-term colorectal cancer survivors: a population-based analysis using the SEER-Medicare healthcare outcomes survey. Support Care Cancer 2016;24(9):3907–14.

72. American College of Surgeons. Cancer program standards: ensuring patient-centered care. Chicago (IL): Commission on Cancer; 2015.

73. Oancea SC, Cheruvu VK. Psychological distress among adult cancer survivors: importance of survivorship care plan. Support Care Cancer 2016;24(11):4523–31.

74. Beutel ME, Fischbeck S, Binder H, et al. Depression, anxiety and quality of life in long-term survivors of malignant melanoma: a register-based cohort study. PLoS One 2015;10(1):e0116440.

75. Benedict C, Rodriguez VM, Carter J, et al. Investigation of body image as a mediator of the effects of bowel and GI symptoms on psychological distress in female survivors of rectal and anal cancer. Support Care Cancer 2016;24(4):1795–802.

76. Begovic-Juhant A, Chmielewski A, Iwuagwu S, et al. Impact of body image on depression and quality of life among women with breast cancer. J Psychosoc Oncol 2012;30(4):446–60.

77. Chongpison Y, Hornbrook MC, Harris RB, et al. Self-reported depression and perceived financial burden among long-term rectal cancer survivors. Psychooncology 2016;25(11):1350–6.

78. Hall AE, Sanson-Fisher RW, Carey ML, et al. Prevalence and associates of psychological distress in haematological cancer survivors. Support Care Cancer 2016;24(10):4413–22.

79. Stanton AL. Psychosocial concerns and interventions for cancer survivors. J Clin Oncol 2006;24(32):5132–7.

80. Marroquin B, Czamanski-Cohen J, Weihs KL, et al. Implicit loneliness, emotion regulation, and depressive symptoms in breast cancer survivors. J Behav Med 2016;39(5):832–44.

81. Avis NE, Levine BJ, Case LD, et al. Trajectories of depressive symptoms following breast cancer diagnosis. Cancer Epidemiol Biomarkers Prev 2015;24(11):1789–95.

82. Brothers BM, Yang HC, Strunk DR, et al. Cancer patients with major depressive disorder: testing a biobehavioral/cognitive behavior intervention. J Consult Clin Psychol 2011;79(2):253–60.

83. Jassim GA, Whitford DL, Hickey A, et al. Psychological interventions for women with non-metastatic breast cancer. Cochrane Database Syst Rev 2015;(5):CD008729.

84. DuHamel KN, Mosher CE, Winkel G, et al. Randomized clinical trial of telephone-administered cognitive-behavioral therapy to reduce post-traumatic stress disorder and distress symptoms after hematopoietic stem-cell transplantation. J Clin Oncol 2010;28(23):3754–61.

85. Carlson LE, Tamagawa R, Stephen J, et al. Randomized-controlled trial of mindfulness-based cancer recovery versus supportive expressive group therapy among distressed breast cancer survivors (MINDSET): long-term follow-up results. Psychooncology 2016;25(7):750–9.

86. Dawson G, Madsen LT, Dains JE. Interventions to manage uncertainty and fear of recurrence in female breast cancer survivors: a review of the literature. Clin J Oncol Nurs 2016;20(6):E155–61.

87. Johns SA, Brown LF, Beck-Coon K, et al. Randomized controlled pilot trial of mindfulness-based stress reduction compared to psychoeducational support for persistently fatigued breast and colorectal cancer survivors. Support Care Cancer 2016;24(10):4085–96.

88. Lengacher CA, Reich RR, Paterson CL, et al. Examination of broad symptom improvement resulting from mindfulness-based stress reduction in breast cancer survivors: a randomized controlled trial. J Clin Oncol 2016;34(24):2827–34.

89. Reich RR, Lengacher CA, Alinat CB, et al. Mindfulness-based stress reduction in post-treatment breast cancer patients: immediate and sustained effects across multiple symptom clusters. J Pain Symptom Manage 2017;53(1):85–95.

90. Johnson AJ, Marcus J, Hickman K, et al. Anxiety reduction among breast-cancer survivors receiving hypnotic relaxation therapy for hot flashes. Int J Clin Exp Hypn 2016;64(4):377–90.

91. van den Berg SW, Gielissen MF, Custers JA, et al. BREATH: web-based self-management for psychological adjustment after primary breast cancer–results of a multicenter randomized controlled trial. J Clin Oncol 2015;33(25):2763–71.

92. Kanera IM, Willems RA, Bolman CA, et al. Use and appreciation of a tailored self-management eHealth intervention for early cancer survivors: process evaluation of a randomized controlled trial. J Med Internet Res 2016;18(8):e229.

93. Kim AR, Park HA. Web-based self-management support interventions for cancer survivors: a systematic review and meta-analyses. Stud Health Technol Inform 2015;216:142–7.

94. Otto AK, Szczesny EC, Soriano EC, et al. Effects of a randomized gratitude intervention on death-related fear of recurrence in breast cancer survivors. Health Psychol 2016;35(12):1320–8.

95. Post KE, Flanagan J. Web based survivorship interventions for women with breast cancer: An integrative review. Eur J Oncol Nurs 2016;25:90–9.

96. Short CE, Rebar A, James EL, et al. How do different delivery schedules of tailored web-based physical activity advice for breast cancer survivors influence intervention use and efficacy? J Cancer Surviv 2017;11(1):80–91.

97. Smith SK, O'Donnell JD, Abernethy AP, et al. Evaluation of Pillars4life: a virtual coping skills program for cancer survivors. Psychooncology 2015;24(11):1407–15.

98. Owen J, Bantum E, Stanton A. Engagement with a social networking intervention for cancer-related distress. Ann Behav Med 2015;49(2):154–64.

99. Cleary EH, Stanton AL. Mediators of an Internet-based psychosocial intervention for women with breast cancer. Health Psychol 2015;34(5):477–85.

100. Okuyama S, Jones W, Ricklefs C, et al. Psychosocial telephone interventions for patients with cancer and survivors: a systematic review. Psychooncology 2015;24(8):857–70.

101. Wenzel L, Osann K, Hsieh S, et al. Psychosocial telephone counseling for survivors of cervical cancer: results of a randomized biobehavioral trial. J Clin Oncol 2015;33(10):1171–9.

102. Zhu G, Zhang X, Wang Y, et al. Effects of exercise intervention in breast cancer survivors: a meta-analysis of 33 randomized controlled trails. Onco Targets Ther 2016;9:2153–68.
103. Gaskin CJ, Craike M, Mohebbi M, et al. A clinician referral and 12-week exercise training programme for men with prostate cancer: outcomes to 12 months of the ENGAGE cluster randomised controlled trial. J Phys Act Health 2017;14(5): 353–9.
104. Biglia N, Bounous VE, Susini T, et al. Duloxetine and escitalopram for hot flushes: efficacy and compliance in breast cancer survivors. Eur J Cancer Care (Engl) 2016. [Epub ahead of print].
105. Haque R, Shi J, Schottinger JE, et al. Tamoxifen and antidepressant drug interaction in a cohort of 16,887 breast cancer survivors. J Natl Cancer Inst 2016; 108(3).
106. Lavigne JE, Heckler C, Mathews JL, et al. A randomized, controlled, double-blinded clinical trial of gabapentin 300 versus 900 mg versus placebo for anxiety symptoms in breast cancer survivors. Breast Cancer Res Treat 2012;136(2): 479–86.
107. Lu D, Andersson TM, Fall K, et al. Clinical diagnosis of mental disorders immediately before and after cancer diagnosis: a Nationwide Matched Cohort Study in Sweden. JAMA Oncol 2016;2(9):1188–96.
108. Simonelli LE, Siegel SD, Duffy NM. Fear of cancer recurrence: a theoretical review and its relevance for clinical presentation and management. Psychooncology 2016. [Epub ahead of print].
109. Stanton AL, Rowland JH, Ganz PA. Life after diagnosis and treatment of cancer in adulthood: contributions from psychosocial oncology research. Am Psychol 2015;70(2):159–74.

Cognitive Changes Related to Cancer Therapy

Tracy D. Vannorsdall, PhD[a,b,]*

KEYWORDS

- Cancer • Cancer-related cognitive impairment • Chemo brain • Chemo fog
- Cognition • Neuropsychological functioning

KEY POINTS

- Cognitive dysfunction is one of the most bothersome symptoms experienced by cancer survivors and is associated with poorer adherence, role functioning, and quality of life.
- Patients commonly show modest impairments in attention, processing speed, executive functioning, and memory that are largely independent of mood, fatigue, and disease status.
- Cognitive impairments are most common during treatment. Patients typically return to baseline within 6 months to 2 years post-treatment, although nearly one-third experience persistent cognitive dysfunction.
- Accurate assessment is crucial for developing effective interventions. Cognitive screening measures, self-report instruments, and neuropsychological evaluation may each be of benefit in guiding treatment.
- Evidence largely supports the use of compensatory strategies, cognitive rehabilitation, and exercise to improve cognition. Brain training and pharmacologic interventions enjoy less empirical support.

INTRODUCTION

It is estimated that more than 1 in 3 individuals will be diagnosed with cancer over their lifetimes.[1] Advances in treatment have resulted in a growing population of cancer survivors; there are currently 15.5 million cancer survivors in the United States.[2] With this growth comes an increased appreciation for the long-term consequences of cancer on the cognitive functioning and quality of life. An ever-growing body of research now demonstrates that a substantial proportion of cancer survivors are at risk for

No disclosures.
[a] Department of Psychiatry and Behavioral Sciences, The Johns Hopkins University School of Medicine, 600 North Wolfe Street, Meyer 218, Baltimore, MD 21287, USA; [b] Department of Neurology, The Johns Hopkins University School of Medicine, 600 North Wolfe Street, Meyer 218, Baltimore, MD 21287, USA
* 600 North Wolfe Street, Meyer 218, Baltimore, MD 21287.
E-mail address: TVannor1@jhmi.edu

medical.theclinics.com

experiencing acute and long-term cognitive consequences of their cancer and its treatment. This article outlines the current state of knowledge regarding cognitive changes in adults treated for non–central nervous system (CNS) cancers.

It is not uncommon for patients to report cognitive difficulties at some point in the course of their disease and treatment. Although cognitive consequences of CNS cancers have been well appreciated for some time, it was long believed that non-CNS cancers did not result in measurable changes in cognition. In part, this assumption stemmed from the belief that chemotherapy was not directly neurotoxic, because it was not thought to cross the blood-brain barrier.[3] As such, patient complaints were often ascribed to stress, anxiety, mood, and other factors. As the scientific study of cancer-related cognitive impairment (CRCI) has advanced over the past more than 20 years, however, evidence supporting the presence of cognitive dysfunction during the course of cancer treatment and survivorship has grown exponentially. Cross-sectional and longitudinal studies of various therapies have been accompanied by advances in translational and neuroimaging work demonstrating potential mechanisms by which cancer and its treatment contribute to CRCI.

The exploration of cognitive decline after the diagnosis of non-CNS cancers has largely focused on the presentation, rates, and consequences of CRCI in women with breast cancer,[4,5] because this is a commonly occurring cancer whose patient population has experienced a surge in improved outcomes over recent decades. That is not to say that that CRCI is exclusive to breast cancer. Although less comprehensively studied, there is growing evidence documenting cognitive changes in patients with colorectal, ovarian, prostate, testicular, and various blood cancers, including lymphoma and multiple myeloma, among others (**Box 1** has a nonexhaustive list of non-CNS cancers associated with CRCI).

THE IMPORTANCE OF NOMENCLATURE

When patients experience cognitive difficulties, they tend to convey a sense of cognitive inefficiency. Patients often describe this in terms of "chemobrain."[6] Although the term has stimulated research and given providers a framework with which to address

---

Box 1
Non–central nervous system cancers with documented links to cancer-related cognitive impairment

Breast

Colorectal

Head and neck

Leukemia

Lung

Lymphoma

Multiple myeloma

Ovarian

Prostate

Skin

Testicular

the issue of cognitive change during and after treatment, the term itself is a misnomer that serves to attribute cognitive alterations to a single, specific cause. Research has shown that cognitive changes experienced by cancer patients may be attributable to several factors, including chemotherapy, radiation, hormonal treatments, surgery, anesthesia, pain, fatigue, medications, and other contributors[7–9] (**Fig. 1**). Cognitive dysfunction has also been demonstrated in patients who have not received chemotherapy.[10] Given this knowledge, the field has adopted the term, *CRCI*.[11] This modification has helped shift appreciation regarding the complexity of the phenomenon as well as spur further research into mechanisms and risk factors associated with cognitive changes in the cancer setting. The term is also preferred because it provides a more empowering message to patients. Namely, although they may realistically have limited control over some aspects of their disease and treatment course, there remain modifiable factors that can be addressed to help minimize cognitive declines and improve quality of life.

AFFECTED COGNITIVE DOMAINS

Patients can experience a variety of changes in thinking across the course of treatment and survivorship. They may complain that it takes them longer to understand and learn new material, and they may find that their ability to retain newly learned

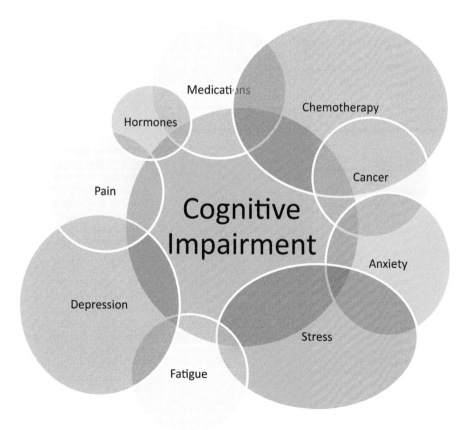

Fig. 1. Potential contributors to CRCI.

information is diminished relative to their preillness abilities. These problems with acquiring and retaining information can be compounded by slowed thinking speed and concentration difficulties that limit patients' attentional resources. Patients also complain of frequent forgetfulness; they may inadvertently miss meetings, misplace or forget needed items, or experience problems retrieving names and words. Also common are problems with multitasking, wherein switching between tasks results in errors and memory problems.

The experience of cognitive change may be different for different patients and across different phases of treatment and survivorship. Although the specific types of cognitive abilities that are most sensitive to cancer and its treatment tend to fluctuate to some degree across investigations, the preponderance of evidence suggests deficits in the domains of learning and memory, attention, processing speed, and executive functioning (**Table 1**). The severity of these changes is generally mild to moderate in non-CNS cancers, particularly compared with the magnitude of change that typically accompanies neurologic disorders, such as stroke or neurodegenerative disease. Nonetheless, such changes may be noticeable to patients and particularly bothersome for those on the ends of the ability spectrum; high-functioning individuals who rely on their intellect and cognitive proficiency for their work may perceive functional declines as a result of little diminution of their skills whereas those with less native ability may find that even minor worsening of their thinking pushes them beyond their capacity to effectively navigate everyday challenges.

CONSEQUENCES OF COGNITIVE CHANGES

The importance of cognition on patient functioning has only recently come into focus as a significant area of concern for both patients and providers. Persistent cognitive

Table 1
Cognitive domains commonly affected in cancer-related cognitive impairment

Cognitive Domain	Definition	Cancer-related Cognitive Impairment Presentation
Attention and working memory	Focused awareness on a select subset of perceptual information; very short-term memory used for immediate conscious processing	Patients with CRCI may describe "spacing out" or difficulty concentrating or multitasking as well as difficulty remembering phone numbers, lists, or names
Processing speed	The ability to automatically and fluently perform simple motor and cognitive tasks; a measure of cognitive efficiency	Patients may describe taking longer to process new information and finish familiar tasks
Executive functioning	Command and control of all cognitive skills; a sort of conductor of general processes	Patients may describe trouble multitasking, planning, and organizing
Learning and memory	Ability to acquire, retain, and efficiently retrieve new information	Patients may describe trouble learning new material, forgetting names or events, or problems "finding" the right word

dysfunction is rated as one of the most bothersome post-treatment symptoms experienced by cancer survivors.[12] In cross-sectional surveys, more than 75% of adult cancer survivors reported cognitive impairment 6 months after treatment,[12] and more than 4 years post-treatment nearly half reported that they viewed their cognition as worse than healthy same-aged peers.[13]

Cognitive dysfunction during and after treatment can have a substantial influence on patient quality of life. During treatment, reduced cognition can contribute to poorer treatment adherence[14] and, therefore, has the potential to affect patient outcomes. As patients transition from active treatment and back to their former roles, they often report that lingering cognitive changes continue to affect their daily life and functioning.[12] Particularly noticeable are changes in social functioning and community involvement. Because cognitive changes are not physically apparent to outside observers, discrepancies between former and current thinking skills and competencies can lead to stress in interpersonal relationships as well as social embarrassment that may serve to isolate patients from their support system, communities, and healthful leisure activities.[15] CRCI also has occupational ramifications and may lead patients to return to work in only a limited capacity.[16] Declines in thinking skills are cited as one of the reasons 13% of cancer survivors drop out of the workforce within 4 years of their diagnosis.[17]

TRAJECTORY
Pretreatment

One of the most striking findings in the study of CRCI comes from longitudinal studies demonstrating that cognitive difficulties can arise at any point over the disease course and are common even prior to treatment onset. When compared with well-matched noncancer controls, approximately 20% to 40% of cancer patients show cognitive deficits at the time of diagnosis, prior to the initiation of any systemic therapies[18,19] (**Fig. 2**). Because the initial postdiagnosis period is often stressful, it might be expected that these cognitive weaknesses are attributable to emotional distress, anxiety, mood problems, or fatigue. Research has repeatedly shown, however, pretreatment cognitive impairment as indexed by objective neuropsychological testing is largely independent of emotional factors and seems generally unrelated to surgical factors and co-occurring medical conditions.[20,21]

Multiple neuroimaging studies have demonstrated structural and functional brain differences between cancer patients and healthy controls that predate systemic treatment, with frontal brain regions critical for attention, executive functioning, and new learning typically affected. For example, Menning and colleagues[10] demonstrated that groups of breast cancer patients who were scheduled to receive chemotherapy and those who were not both performed worse on cognitive testing when compared with a no-cancer control group. They also demonstrated prefrontal hyperactivation in response to an increasingly difficult planning task and reduced white matter integrity.

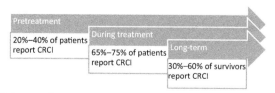

Pretreatment
20%–40% of patients report CRCI

During treatment
65%–75% of patients report CRCI

Long-term
30%–60% of survivors report CRCI

Fig. 2. Rates of CRCI over time.

Increased hyperactivation is thought to reflect a compensatory mechanism by increasing neural resources required to successfully perform a task. Decreased white matter integrity may reflect poorer neuronal transmission.

Clinically, the consistency with which studies document the presence of early, pre-treatment cognitive deficits suggests that early cognitive deficits are common in a subset of patients. Given the functional consequences of CRCI, formal cognitive assessment may be appropriate for select patients directly after diagnosis. This type of assessment could help identify CRCI and allow the initiation of strategies to mitigate cognitive and functional deficits in patients who are concerned about the possibility of experiencing cognitive changes throughout the course of their treatment or who may be at risk of functional declines associated with changes in their thinking.

Active Treatment

The bulk of well-designed longitudinal studies demonstrate that approximately 65% to 75% of patients experience demonstrable cognitive declines during and very soon after the termination of cancer treatment.[5,6,19]

Post-treatment

The rates of cognitive impairment tend to stabilize within the first 6 months and are often followed by a 1-year to 2-year recovery process in affected individuals.[22,23] Although it is often reported that approximately one-third of patients show persistent cognitive deficits a year or so post-treatment,[24] some studies suggest higher rates as well as new-onset cognitive dysfunction in the ensuing post-treatment years. For example, in Wefel and colleagues'[19] longitudinal study of breast cancer survivors, more than 60% evidenced cognitive impairment at 1-year post-treatment and a full 61% of these cases represented new-onset deficits in patients who did not previously meet criteria for CRCI.

The finding of persistent and later-onset cognitive dysfunction has raised questions about the long-term cognitive functioning of cancer survivors. Although most longitudinal research on adult-onset non-CNS cancers has focused on the first few years after treatment, studies are increasingly exploring outcomes over longer survival periods. Most find greater than expected rates of impairment 5 years to 21 years post-diagnosis.[25] Attention and executive functioning are the most frequently impaired domains across studies, although some studies also suggest a persistent risk of long-term memory dysfunction in a subset of patients.

Post-treatment cognitive changes have repeatedly been shown associated with both brain alterations occurring as early as 1-month post-treatment and persisting for as long as 2 decades. Changes in both brain structure and function have been demonstrated in terms of gray matter volume loss,[26,27] reduced white matter integrity,[27,28] overactivation of frontal regions in response to cognitive challenges,[29] and altered cerebral network organization.[30] These brain changes are often associated with subjective and/or objective cognitive deficits and may help explain the presence of persistent cognitive weakness in a subset of cancer survivors.

Cancer History as a Risk Factor for Dementia

Given that longitudinal studies suggest a proportion of survivors are likely to experience persistent, modest cognitive difficulties for decades after their treatment, patients often express concern about whether their cancer history puts them at increased risk for developing dementia later in life. Here the data are generally reassuring. Several large epidemiologic studies have shown that cancer survivors are generally at decreased risk of developing Alzheimer disease. Data from the Framingham

Heart Study documented that over 10 years, cancer survivors had a 33% reduced risk of developing Alzheimer disease relative to those with no such history.[31] Similarly, a northern Italian study found the risk of developing Alzheimer disease was reduced by 35% in cancer patients whereas the risk of developing cancer was reduced by 50% in those with an Alzheimer diagnosis.[32] Data from the Cardiovascular Health Study suggest that the protective effect of a cancer history seems to pertain specifically to Alzheimer dementia and not to vascular or mixed forms of neurodegenerative disease.[33]

Although there remains much to be learned about the potential risk of specific cancer treatments and later dementia outcomes, several studies have compared dementia rates in chemotherapy-exposed and chemotherapy-nonexposed breast cancer survivors. One study found that dementia diagnoses were more common in chemotherapy-exposed survivors,[34] whereas others demonstrated that for older women (aged 76–80) chemotherapy exposure was related to reduced dementia risk and there was no chemotherapy-dementia link in younger age cohorts.[35] Du and colleagues[36] showed that once tumor and patient characteristics are accounted for, the risk of both vascular and Alzheimer dementia is reduced in chemotherapy-exposed survivors compared with those who did not receive chemotherapy. There is also no evidence for differential risk of later dementia based on type of cytotoxic agent regimen.[37]

RISK FACTORS FOR CANCER-RELATED COGNITIVE IMPAIRMENT

There are several factors that may predispose or perpetuate cognitive dysfunction in a subset of cancer patients. These factors range from largely immutable to those that are more amenable to intervention by patients and/or their treatment team (**Fig. 3**).

Genetics and Molecular Risks

There are several genetic polymorphisms that have been linked to CRCI severity, although more work is needed to confirm these initial findings. Apolipoprotein E plays a key role in neuronal repair, is associated with a range of cognitive conditions, and is the strongest single genetic risk factor for Alzheimer disease. Cancer survivors with at least 1 E4 allele have been shown to exhibit worse cognition than survivors without an E4 allele.[38] Single-nucleotide polymorphisms in catechol-O-methyltransferase (COMT) are associated with prefrontal cortex dopamine levels and associated cognitive skills. Methionine carriers tend to show reduced dopamine degradation relative to Valine carriers. COMT Met carriers also perform better on cognitive testing[39] and report fewer subjective cognitive complaints than their Val-carrying counterparts when both groups have been exposed to chemotherapy.[40]

Chemotherapy has been associated with increased proinflammatory cytokines.[3,5,41] Increased cytokine levels correlate with reduced cognitive functioning[42] as well as the degree of structural and functional brain changes observed in cancer

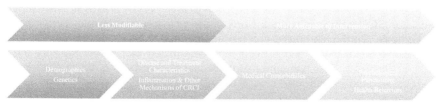

Fig. 3. Risk factors associated with CRCI.

patients.[26] Other suspected potentiators of CRCI include cancer-related and treatment-related neurogenesis, changes in blood flow and the integrity of the blood-brain barrier, neurogenesis, oxidative stress, and hypothalamic-pituitary-adrenal axis functioning as well as DNA damage and damage to DNA repair mechanisms.[43]

Demographics

Although both older and younger adults experience CRCI, most research has been conducted in patients under the age of 60. Nonetheless, some evidence suggests a particular vulnerability to cognitive decline among elderly patients diagnosed with cancer.[22,44] Similarly, the bulk of CRCI research has been conducted in women with breast cancer. There is some evidence that cognitive dysfunction occurs at greater rates in women versus men who have been treated for cancer,[45,46] but it is apparent that men also experience cancer-related and treatment-related changes in their thinking and functioning.[47] Cognitive reserve refers to the variability across individuals with respect to a person's susceptibility to age-related and pathology-related brain changes. Often indexed by preillness IQ or years of educational attainment, cognitive reserve is thought to mediate the relationship between the degree of cerebral insult and the degree to which cognitive dysfunction is manifested clinically.[48] There is some evidence that lower cognitive reserve puts cancer patients at increased risk of experiencing treatment-related dysfunction.[22] Other demographic factors, such as race, ethnicity, and socioeconomic status, have yet to be examined as they pertain to CRCI risk.

Specific Treatments

There has been disappointingly little work examining the relative toxicity profiles of various chemotherapeutic agents. A 2013 meta-analysis found evidence for poorer cognitive outcomes with more prolonged treatment.[49] There is also evidence for a dose-response relationship between chemotherapy intensity and the severity of CRCI as documented in both breast[50] and testicular cancers.[47] Furthermore, the potential for acute neurologic complications including encephalopathies is present in association with some agents, including methotrexate, bevacizumab, carmustine, melphalan, fludarabine, cytarabine, 5-fluorouracil, levamisole, cisplatin, and capecitabine.[51–54] Although anthracyclines are generally considered more neurotoxic than nonanthracyclines,[44] a recent large, prospective, nationwide study of women receiving treatment of breast cancer found no difference in self-reported cognitive dysfunction up to 6 months after treatment based on treatment type.[55]

Hormone therapies work via the blocking of sex hormone production or suppressing of hormone receptors to reduce or inhibit tumor growth. Such treatments are often proscribed for prolonged periods in those with breast or prostate cancer and they are associated with side effects that include changes in mood, hot flashes, and fatigue. Both estrogen and androgen receptors are widely distributed in the cerebral cortex and hippocampus, and thus there is concern that these agents may exert bothersome cognitive side effects.

Several recent meta-analytic studies and reviews have been conducted examining short-term (<2 years) and longer-term (>2 years) use of the selective estrogen receptor modulator (SERM) tamoxifen and the aromatase inhibitors anastrozole, exemestane, and letrozole. Both meta-analyses noted that methodological issues preclude clear conclusions. Bakoyiannis and colleagues[56] determined that verbal memory most frequently changed after hormone treatment, but the direction of these differences varied across studies with some studies showing improved verbal memory and others showing declines. Overall they found a trend toward better cognition with aromatase inhibitors over SERMs. Lee's recent meta-analysis[57] found than 80% of studies demonstrated cognitive impairment associated with hormone therapies, but the cognitive domains differed widely across studies, there were no clear patterns found between different therapy regimens, and the cognitive effects of hormone therapy did not differ from chemotherapy, suggesting that some individuals may be prone to CRCI irrespective of the specific treatment received. Finally, a review by Zwart and colleagues[58] suggested evidence for cognitive effects of SERMs, but there were no conclusive findings regarding the cognitive effects of aromatase inhibitors.

Androgen deprivation therapy (ADT) can include luteinizing hormone–releasing hormone agonists (gonadotropin-releasing hormone agonists), luteinizing hormone–releasing hormone antagonists, and oral antiandrogens (eg, bicalutamide and flutamide). Early reviews tended to show cognitive dysfunction after the initiation of ADT, but these reviews were of uniformly low quality.[59] A more recent high-quality review by McGinty and colleagues[60] concluded that patients on ADT showed significantly poorer visuospatial reasoning and visuomotor functioning compared with controls, which is consistent with the known cognitive effects of testosterone.

Lifestyle and Noncancer Medical Factors

Lifestyle and medical comorbidities may contribute to CRCI but have generally not been found to be robust predictors of cognitive dysfunction.[4,19,61] Some research suggests, however, that the presence of diabetes and cardiovascular disease is associated with pretreatment cognitive impairment and that the medical comorbidities, when present, are linked to greater rates of CRCI, specifically in the elderly.[61] Similarly, surgical factors and effects of anesthesia have been hypothesized to be potential contributors to CRCI, but the evidence is not compelling.[62] Other factors, such as menopause status and disease stage, as well more modifiable factors, such as nutrition and body mass index, have yet to be carefully investigated as potential contributors to CRCI.

Distress and Associated Symptoms

Affective symptoms, such as depression and anxiety as well as fatigue, are common throughout the course of cancer diagnosis, treatment, and survivorship. It is well known that these symptoms can exert significant deleterious impact on cognitive efficiency. Unlike genetic, demographic, and many medical risk factors for CRCI, mood and fatigue represent largely modifiable risk factors and reflect potential targets for intervention. Some individuals may be at heightened risk for clinically significant distress, including those with a history of mental illness, younger patients, and those facing other life stressors, including low socioeconomic status or unemployment.[63] In 2015 the American Cancer Society/American Society of Clinical Oncology issued survivorship care guidelines that, although geared toward breast cancer patients, may be applicable to those caring for patients with a variety of non-CNS cancers.[64]

Cognitive profiles characteristic of depression and anxiety often include psychomotor slowing, inefficient learning, and executive dysfunction, all of which are commonly reported features of CRCI. Research generally shows that affective distress, including scores on formal measures of depressive symptomatology and anxiety correlate more robustly with subjective patient ratings of cognitive dysfunction than with cognitive functioning as objectively measured on formal neuropsychological tests.[65] Given the critical role depression and anxiety play in perceived cognitive dysfunction and patient quality of life, treatment of these issues has the potential to substantially improve the patient experience. As discussed later and elsewhere in this series, psychiatric disorders are amenable to standard treatments in cancer patients. Hence, although distress and a period of emotional adjustment are common and not necessarily pathologic after a cancer diagnosis, clinically significant depression and anxiety should not be considered an expected result of a stressful medical condition and warrant targeted intervention.

Fatigue is a common symptom that frequently accompanies anxiety and depression, which also has strong links to cognitive functioning in cancer patients and survivors.[66] As with depression and anxiety, subjective fatigue is more closely linked to perceived rather than objectively measured cognitive dysfunction.[67] Research has begun to explore whether fatigue's link to cognition represents a psychological or neurologic basis for cognitive impairment in cancer patients, with more recent evidence pointing to the latter. Because subjective cognitive dysfunction tends to show more robust or consistent relationships with functional brain changes seen on neuroimaging,[10] it is hypothesized that the increased, compensatory neural activation required to perform cognitive tasks is itself fatiguing and may underlie patient perceptions of both cognitive fatigue and dysfunction.[68]

SPECIAL POPULATIONS
Adult Survivors of Childhood Cancers

Survivors of childhood cancers are at elevated risk for a range of mental health problems and cognitive dysfunction. Treatments, such as cranial irradiation, have long been known to negatively affect children's IQ[69] and may interact with chemotherapies and other treatments to impair other aspects of cognition over the long term. Large cohort studies have found that approximately half of all survivors of pediatric cancers demonstrate objective cognitive difficulties in adulthood.[70] Similar to the deficits seen in cancers of adulthood, cognitive dysfunction typically occurs in relation to attention, processing speed, executive functioning, and memory.[71] Risk factors for cognitive dysfunction in children include female gender, cranial irradiation, hearing impairment, and the receipt of treatment before age 6.[72] Although younger age at treatment is an established risk factor, newer work suggests that those treated in early adolescence or early young adulthood (ages 11–21) are also at risk for poorer outcomes. These individuals experience problems with emotional regulation and demonstrate greater rates of depression and anxiety. They also show deficits is executive functioning and memory and are at greater risk for poor functional outcomes, such as unemployment.[73]

New-Onset Cancer in the Elderly

A majority of new cancers occur in the growing population of adults age 65 or older,[1] yet few studies have focused on CRCI in older adults. As part of the normal aging process, most elderly experience declines in processing speed, attention, aspects of executive functioning, and memory. They are also at increased risk for dementia, medical comorbidities that contribute to cognitive dysfunction (eg, hypertension and diabetes), the use of medications with potential cognitive side effects, and both mood and anxiety disorders. Hence, for many older adults, the onset and treatment of cancer reflect additional risks for cognitive dysfunction within the context of an already vulnerable system. Some evidence suggests that older patients with localized cancers exhibit greater rates of baseline cognitive dysfunction than is seen in younger cohorts.[44]

Those studies that have focused on older, nondemented patients document a prevalence rate of cognitive dysfunction in up to half of patients,[74] with alterations generally occurring in the same cognitive domains as seen in younger adults (ie, attention, processing speed, memory, and executive functioning). As with their younger peers, cognitive changes seem to persist in a subset of older patients.[44] Although a history of cancer during early life or midlife does not necessarily increase risk of developing dementia, less is known about the role of cancer and its treatment as potential precipitators of dementia when first diagnosed in older adulthood. What has been well documented is that those developing cancer in the context of a preexisting dementia have increased risk of mortality from noncancer causes than their nondemented counterparts.[75] Older adults with mild cognitive impairment but not dementia at cancer onset are also up to 6 times more likely to die in the 2 years after treatment, with baseline cognition serving as a more powerful predictor of mortality than loss of instrumental autonomy or fatigue.[76]

ASSESSMENT

Accurately assessing patient cognitive and psychological functioning is a crucial step in developing and implementing effective interventions and treatment plans. Assessment tools fall into 2 broad categories: objective measures of cognition and patient-reported outcomes/self-report measures. There is much to be gained from each approach. Subjective cognitive complaints often do not correspond to objectively assessed cognitive ability. Patients may not be aware of how their thinking has changed and how these changes negatively affect functioning. Objective test results bring such issues to light and can guide practical remediation strategies. Subjective cognitive complaints are no less real or functionally limiting. Given that studies have repeatedly shown patient perceptions of their cognition correlates more strongly with affective distress and fatigue, this suggests these may be more appropriate intervention targets for some patients.

There are several brief assessment tools available to practitioners that can serve to guide interventions or alert the treatment team to the need for a more formal cognitive workup (**Table 2**). The most commonly used objective screening tools include the Montreal Cognitive Assessment (MoCA)[77] and the Mini-Mental State Examination (MMSE).[78] Unfortunately, cognitive screening measures, such as these, lack the sensitivity to detect subtle changes in cognition and are generally considered insufficient for detecting CRCI. Nonetheless, they may be of some utility; although passing a cognitive screening measure does not rule out the presence of CRCI, a patient performing near or below cutoffs for impairment suggests that a formal assessment via referral to a neuropsychologist may be useful. There are numerous self-report measures of cognitive complaints specifically designed for cancer patients (eg, the Functional Assessment of Cancer Therapy–Cognitive Function [FACT-Cog][79]). These may be helpful in detecting clinically significant cognitive complaints. Because subjective cognitive functioning is so tightly linked with depression, anxiety, and fatigue, however, administration of mood symptom questionnaires may be more useful than subjective cognitive screening measures in patients with cognitive concerns.

Neuropsychological assessment is considered the gold standard in detecting CRCI.[80] Conducted by a doctoral-level psychologist, neuropsychological assessment involves a review of medical records, detailed interview with the patient and informants, completion of psychometrically sound paper-and-pencil neuropsychological tests assessing a range of cognitive domains, and the completion of self-report questionnaires addressing mood, symptoms, and functioning. Cognitive test scores are compared with healthy samples of individuals of similar demographic (age, gender, and ethnicity), educational, and sometimes intellectual backgrounds to determine a patient's current areas of strength and weakness. This information provides concrete data on which compensatory strategies and treatment interventions can be tailored and against which change can be measured. Neuropsychological evaluation also

Table 2
Common cognitive screening and symptom self-report measures

Measure	Assessed	Administration	Scores and Cutoffs	Availability
MoCA[77]	Executive functioning Visuoconstruction Language Memory Attention Orientation	Examiner-administered 5–10 min	0-30 (+1 point if education ≤12 y) ≥26/30 (normal)	Free of charge at http://www.mocatest.org
MMSE[78]	Orientation Registration Attention/calculation Language Memory Visuoconstruction	Examiner-administered 5–10 min	0-30 ≥24/30 (normal)	Licensed and published by Psychological Assessment Resources
FACT-Cog[79]	Frequency of cognitive symptoms over the past week 6 domains: Memory Concentration Mental acuity Verbal fluency Functional interference Multitasking Subscales: Noticeability Quality of life Total score	Self-report 37-item Likert scale response format 5–10 min	0-148 Higher scores reflect better functioning	Free of charge for clinical use at http://www.facit.org/FACITOrg

Data from Refs.[77–79]

identifies modifiable contributors to cognitive and emotional dysfunction and helps address them via the facilitation of treatment of mood disorders and substance abuse, pain management, sleep hygiene training, and other interventions. Results of neuropsychological evaluation can also be used to help identify academic and workplace accommodations that may facilitate a patient's successful return to former roles.

INTERVENTIONS

A range of interventions strategies is available to help minimize cognitive dysfunction in patients with non-CNS cancers (**Box 2**). These vary from less to more invasive and in terms of their intensity and duration. The breadth of empirically supported intervention strategies available to cancer patients indicates that there are multiple pathways to improve patient cognition and functioning. Choosing the most appropriate intervention for a given patient should be a collaborative exercise between the patient and provider, taking the patient's unique circumstances and preferences as well as practical matters, such as availability and insurance coverage, into account.

Nonpharmacologic Strategies

Psychoeducation

Patients with concerns about their thinking may benefit from learning about the rates and course of CRCI. Simply informing patients that their treatment is associated with potential cognitive side effects, however, can place them at increased risk for later cognitive complaints.[81] Thus, it is important to frame this information in an accurate light that sets the stage optimistic expectations, highlighting that only a subset of patients experience CRCI and, although it can be bothersome, these changes are generally mild and are expected to resolve in the months and years after treatment for most patients.

Behavioral strategies

Once a patient's cognitive strengths and weakness are clarified either through a detailed discussion of difficulties or formal neuropsychological evaluation, a range of compensatory strategies can be generated. Compensatory strategies have been shown effective.[82] They involve using a patient's existing areas of cognitive strength, at times augmented with assistive tools, to strategically compensate for areas of

Box 2
Interventions
Nonpharmacologic strategies
Psychoeducation
Behavioral/compensatory strategies
Cognitive rehabilitation
Brain training
Physical exercise
Biofeedback
Brain stimulation
Pharmacologic strategies
Psychostimulants
Acetylcholinesterase inhibitors

weaknesses. Often this involves hands-on training and practice of these strategies in real-world situations to help establish their efficacious use and integrate them into patients' everyday functioning.

Cognitive rehabilitation

Formal cognitive rehabilitation programs, most of which were originally developed for use in patients with traumatic brain injury and stroke, have been adapted for use in cancer patients. Rehabilitation programs typically occur as a clinic-based program of individual or group outpatient therapy led by a trained clinician (neuropsychologist, psychologist, occupational therapist, or speech language therapist) with the goal of improving patient cognition and real-world functioning. Studies show generally favorable results for both objective and subjective cognitive outcomes.[4,83] Manualized training programs are also being developed to help facilitate empirically supported, cancer-specific cognitive rehabilitation protocols.[84]

Brain training

Cognitive brain training typically focuses on improving a specific cognitive domain by distributed, adaptive practice of specific skills, often via computerized games or exercises.[4] This approach has the benefits of being accessible (multiple platforms are available commercially), home based, and relatively low cost. Evidence suggests that this approach can be effective at improving the skills that are targeted. There is less evidence, however, that these improvements generalize to other tasks or real-life functioning.

Physical exercise

Physical activity has long been associated with improved cognition, in particular executive functioning. Both animal and human studies document a variety of direct biological mechanisms for exercise's beneficial brain effects, many of which overlap with the suspected pathologic mechanisms of CRCI. Exercise may also indirectly improve cognition by ameliorating the cognitively damaging effects of medical comorbidities, such as obesity, hypertension, and diabetes, as well as psychological comorbidities, such as depression and fatigue. Importantly, research suggests that physical activity need not be either intensive or prolonged in order for patients to experience improvements in subjective and objective cognition and quality of life. For example, interventions, such as yoga, qigong, and tai chi, have produced cognitive benefits in as little as a month.[4]

Biofeedback and brain stimulation

Biofeedback involves providing a patient real-time feedback regarding brain activity to teach self-regulation of brain functioning. It is most commonly facilitated with electroencephalogram, but other implementation methods are being explored. Preliminary evidence suggests promise for this approach.[85] Brain stimulation approaches, such as repeated transcranial magnetic stimulation and transcranial direct current stimulation, have shown positive effects on cognition, mood, and fatigue in other patient populations but have yet to be studied in the context of CRCI.

Pharmacologic Strategies

Several small studies have explored the utility of psychostimulants, such as methylphenidate and modafinil, and the acetylcholinesterase inhibitor donepezil as treatments for CRCI. Results have been conflicting and more work with these agents is needed. A randomized clinical trial did not find any benefit to ginkgo biloba.[86] Preclinical studies are showing promising results for antioxidants for ameliorating cognitive dysfunction,[87] whereas animal studies suggest fluoxetine may be effective at preventing CRCI.[88]

FUTURE CONSIDERATIONS AND SUMMARY

A growing population of cancer survivors is at risk for experiencing poorer functioning and quality of life due to cancer-related cognitive dysfunction. Research has several risk factors and potential mechanisms for the development and persistence of CRCI, but more work is needed to allow for the early identification of patients who may be at heightened risk of cognitive decline associated with their disease and its treatment. There is also a need to better understand the discrepancy between patient-reported cognitive dysfunction and performance as measured on cognitive tests, because subjective and objective deficits are largely unrelated. At present, the most effective interventions include cognitive rehabilitation, physical exercise, and the targeting of psychosocial contributors to cognitive dysfunction. Additional preclinical and translational studies are needed to determine the efficacy of promising pharmacologic interventions to prevent and ameliorate CRCI.

Cognitive dysfunction in the areas of attention, processing speed, executive functioning, and memory are common and can occur at any point in the course of cancer treatment and survivorship. These deficits are typically modest but can have a substantial impact on patient functioning and quality of life. Longitudinal studies suggest that many patients will experience declines in thinking during active treatment but most can expect to return to their prediagnosis baseline within 6 months to 2 years after treatment. For a proportion of patients cognitive dysfunction persists for years or decades. Accurate assessment of a patient's pattern of cognitive strengths and weaknesses as well as identification of psychological and environmental contributors to cognitive decline and distress are essential in guiding the selection of the most appropriate, empirically supported intervention for a given patient.

REFERENCES

1. Howlader N, Noone A, Krapcho M, et al. SEER cancer statistics review, 1975-2013. Bethesda (MD): National Cancer Institute. Available at: http://seer.cancer.gov/csr/1975_2010/. Accessed February 20, 2017.
2. Bluethmann SM, Mariotto AB, Rowland JH. Anticipating the "Silver tsunami": prevalence trajectories and comorbidity burden among older cancer survivors in the United States. Cancer Epidemiol Biomarkers Prev 2016;25(7):1029–36.
3. Ahles TA, Saykin AJ. Candidate mechanisms for chemotherapy-induced cognitive changes. Nat Rev Cancer 2007;7(3):192–201.
4. Wefel JS, Kesler SR, Noll KR, et al. Clinical characteristics, pathophysiology, and management of noncentral nervous system cancer-related cognitive impairment in adults. CA Cancer J Clin 2015;65(2):123–38.
5. Janelsins MC, Kesler SR, Ahles TA, et al. Prevalence, mechanisms, and management of cancer-related cognitive impairment. Int Rev Psychiatry 2014;26(1):102–13.
6. Ouimet LA, Stewart A, Collins B, et al. Measuring neuropsychological change following breast cancer treatment: an analysis of statistical models. J Clin Exp Neuropsychol 2009;31(1):73–89.
7. Castellon SA, Ganz PA, Bower JE, et al. Neurocognitive performance in breast cancer survivors exposed to adjuvant chemotherapy and tamoxifen. J Clin Exp Neuropsychol 2004;26(7):955–69.

8. Schilder CM, Eggens PC, Seynaeve C, et al. Neuropsychological functioning in postmenopausal breast cancer patients treated with tamoxifen or exemestane after AC-chemotherapy: cross-sectional findings from the neuropsychological TEAM-side study. Acta Oncol 2009;48(1):76–85.

9. Schilder CM, Seynaeve C, Beex LV, et al. Effects of tamoxifen and exemestane on cognitive functioning of postmenopausal patients with breast cancer: results from the neuropsychological side study of the tamoxifen and exemestane adjuvant multinational trial. J Clin Oncol 2010;28(8):1294–300.

10. Menning S, de Ruiter MB, Veltman DJ, et al. Multimodal MRI and cognitive function in patients with breast cancer prior to adjuvant treatment–the role of fatigue. Neuroimage Clin 2015;7:547–54.

11. Hurria A, Somlo G, Ahles T. Renaming "chemobrain". Cancer Invest 2007;25(6): 373–7.

12. Boykoff N, Moieni M, Subramanian SK. Confronting chemobrain: an in-depth look at survivors' reports of impact on work, social networks, and health care response. J Cancer Surviv 2009;3(4):223–32.

13. Schmidt LH, Kummel A, Gorlich D, et al. PD-1 and PD-L1 Expression in NSCLC indicate a favorable prognosis in defined subgroups. PLoS One 2015;10(8): e0136023.

14. Dos Santos M, Lange M, Clarisse B, et al. Impact of cognitive function on oral anticancer therapies adherence. Ann Oncol 2016;27(6):497–521.

15. Reid-Arndt SA, Yee A, Perry MC, et al. Cognitive and psychological factors associated with early posttreatment functional outcomes in breast cancer survivors. J Psychosoc Oncol 2009;27(4):415–34.

16. Bradley CJ, Neumark D, Bednarek HL, et al. Short-term effects of breast cancer on labor market attachment: results from a longitudinal study. J Health Econ 2005;24(1):137–60.

17. Short PF, Vasey JJ, Tunceli K. Employment pathways in a large cohort of adult cancer survivors. Cancer 2005;103(6):1292–301.

18. Ahles TA. Brain vulnerability to chemotherapy toxicities. Psychooncology 2012; 21(11):1141–8.

19. Wefel JS, Saleeba AK, Buzdar AU, et al. Acute and late onset cognitive dysfunction associated with chemotherapy in women with breast cancer. Cancer 2010; 116(14):3348–56.

20. Wefel JS, Lenzi R, Theriault RL, et al. The cognitive sequelae of standard-dose adjuvant chemotherapy in women with breast carcinoma: results of a prospective, randomized, longitudinal trial. Cancer 2004;100(11):2292–9.

21. Berman M, Askren M, Jung M, et al. Pretreatment worry and neurocognitive responses in women with breast cancer. Health Psychol 2014;33(3):222–31.

22. Ahles TA, Saykin AJ, McDonald BC, et al. Longitudinal assessment of cognitive changes associated with adjuvant treatment for breast cancer: impact of age and cognitive reserve. J Clin Oncol 2010;28(29):4434–40.

23. Schagen SB, Muller MJ, Boogerd W, et al. Late effects of adjuvant chemotherapy on cognitive function: a follow-up study in breast cancer patients. Ann Oncol 2002;13(9):1387–97.

24. Janelsins MC, Kohli S, Mohile SG, et al. An update on cancer- and chemotherapy-related cognitive dysfunction: current status. Semin Oncol 2011; 38(3):431–8.

25. Koppelmans V, Breteler MM, Boogerd W, et al. Late effects of adjuvant chemotherapy for adult onset non-CNS cancer; cognitive impairment, brain structure and risk of dementia. Crit RevOncol Hematol 2013;88(1):87–101.

26. McDonald BC, Conroy SK, Smith DJ, et al. Frontal gray matter reduction after breast cancer chemotherapy and association with executive symptoms: a replication and extension study. Brain Behav Immun 2013;30(Suppl):S117–25.

27. Koppelmans V, de Groot M, de Ruiter MB, et al. Global and focal white matter integrity in breast cancer survivors 20 years after adjuvant chemotherapy. Hum Brain Mapp 2014;35(3):889–99.

28. de Ruiter MB, Reneman L, Boogerd W, et al. Late effects of high-dose adjuvant chemotherapy on white and gray matter in breast cancer survivors: converging results from multimodal magnetic resonance imaging. Hum Brain Mapp 2012; 33(12):2971–83.

29. McDonald BC, Conroy SK, Ahles TA, et al. Alterations in brain activation during working memory processing associated with breast cancer and treatment: a prospective functional magnetic resonance imaging study. J Clin Oncol 2012;30(20): 2500–8.

30. Bruno J, Hosseini SM, Kesler S. Altered resting state functional brain network topology in chemotherapy-treated breast cancer survivors. Neurobiol Dis 2012; 48(3):329–38.

31. Driver JA, Beiser A, Au R, et al. Inverse association between cancer and Alzheimer's disease: results from the Framingham Heart Study. BMJ 2012;344: e1442.

32. Musicco M, Adorni F, Di Santo S, et al. Inverse occurrence of cancer and Alzheimer disease. Neurology 2013;81:322–8.

33. Rao R, Descamps O, John V, et al. Ayurvedic medicinal plants for alzheimers disease: a review. Alzheimers Res Ther 2012;4(3):22.

34. Heck JE, Albert SM, Franco R, et al. Patterns of dementia diagnosis in surveillance, epidemiology, and end results breast cancer survivors who use chemotherapy. J Am Geriatr Soc 2008;56(9):1687–92.

35. Baxter NN, Durham SB, Phillips KA, et al. Risk of dementia in older breast cancer survivors: a population-based cohort study of the association with adjuvant chemotherapy. J Am Geriatr Soc 2009;57(3):403–11.

36. Du XL, Xia R, Hardy D. Relationship between chemotherapy use and cognitive impairments in older women with breast cancer: findings from a large population-based cohort. Am J Clin Oncol 2010;33(6):533–43.

37. Raji MA, Tamborello LP, Kuo YF, et al. Risk of subsequent dementia diagnoses does not vary by types of adjuvant chemotherapy in older women with breast cancer. Med Oncol 2009;26(4):452–9.

38. Ahles TA, Saykin AJ, Noll WW, et al. The relationship of APOE genotype to neuropsychological performance in long-term cancer survivors treated with standard dose chemotherapy. Psychooncology 2003;12(6):612–9.

39. Small BJ, Rawson KS, Walsh E, et al. Catechol-O-methyltransferase genotype modulates cancer treatment-related cognitive deficits in breast cancer survivors. Cancer 2011;117(7):1369–76.

40. Cheng H, Li W, Gan C, et al. The COMT (rs165599) gene polymorphism contributes to chemotherapy-induced cognitive impairment in breast cancer patients. Am J Transl Res 2016;8(11):5087–97.

41. Janelsins MC, Mustian KM, Palesh OG, et al. Differential expression of cytokines in breast cancer patients receiving different chemotherapies: implications for cognitive impairment research. Support Care Cancer 2012;20(4):831–9.

42. Vardy JL, Booth C, Pond GR, et al. Cytokine levels in patients (pts) with colorectal cancer and breast cancer and their relationship to fatigue and cognitive function. Clin Oncol 2007;25(18):9070.

43. Seigers R, Fardell JE. Neurobiological basis of chemotherapy-induced cognitive impairment: a review of rodent research. Neurosci Biobehav Rev 2011;35(3):729–41.
44. Lange M, Giffard B, Noal S, et al. Baseline cognitive functions among elderly patients with localised breast cancer. Eur J Cancer 2014;50(13):2181–9.
45. Heflin LH, Meyerowitz BE, Hall P, et al. Cancer as a risk factor for long-term cognitive deficits and dementia. J Natl Cancer Inst 2005;97(11):854–6.
46. Yamada T, Denburg N, Beglinger L, et al. Neuropsychological outcomes of older breast cancer survivors: cognitive features ten or more years after chemotherapy. J Neuropsychiatry Clin Neurosci 2010;22:48–54.
47. Wefel JS, Vidrine DJ, Marani SK, et al. A prospective study of cognitive function in men with non-seminomatous germ cell tumors. Psychooncology 2014;23(6):626–33.
48. Stern Y. Cognitive reserve in ageing and Alzheimer's disease. Lancet Neurol 2012;11(11):1006–12.
49. Hodgson KD, Hutchinson AD, Wilson CJ, et al. A meta-analysis of the effects of chemotherapy on cognition in patients with cancer. Cancer Treat Rev 2013;39(3):297–304.
50. Collins B, MacKenzie J, Tasca GA, et al. Cognitive effects of chemotherapy in breast cancer patients: a dose-response study. Psychooncology 2013;22(7):1517–27.
51. Chen A, Agarwal N. Reversible posterior leucoencephalopathy syndrome associated with sunitinib. Intern Med J 2009;39(5):341–2.
52. Wefel JS, Schagen SB. Chemotherapy-related cognitive dysfunction. Curr Neurol Neurosci Rep 2012;12(3):267–75.
53. Perry A, Schmidt RE. Cancer therapy-associated CNS neuropathology: an update and review of the literature. Acta Neuropathol 2006;111(3):197–212.
54. Videnovic A, Semenov I, Chua-Adajar R, et al. Capecitabine induced multifocal leukoencephalopathy: a report of five cases. Neurology 2005;65:1792–4.
55. Janelsins MC, Heckler CE, Peppone LJ, et al. Cognitive complaints in survivors of breast cancer after chemotherapy compared with age-matched controls: an analysis from a nationwide, multicenter, prospective longitudinal study. J Clin Oncol 2016. JCO2016685856. [Epub ahead of print].
56. Bakoyiannis I, Tsigka EA, Perrea D, et al. The Impact of endocrine therapy on cognitive functions of breast cancer patients: a systematic review. Clin Drug Investig 2016;36(2):109–18.
57. Lee JH. The effects of music on pain: a meta-analysis. J Music Ther 2016;53(4):430–77.
58. Zwart W, Terra H, Linn SC, et al. Cognitive effects of endocrine therapy for breast cancer: keep calm and carry on? Nat Rev Clin Oncol 2015;12(10):597–606.
59. Wu LM, Amidi A. Cognitive impairment following hormone therapy: current opinion of research in breast and prostate cancer patients. Curr Opin Support Palliat Care 2017;11(1):38–45.
60. McGinty HL, Phillips KM, Jim HS, et al. Cognitive functioning in men receiving androgen deprivation therapy for prostate cancer: a systematic review and meta-analysis. Support Care Cancer 2014;22(8):2271–80.
61. Mandelblatt JS, Stern RA, Luta G, et al. Cognitive impairment in older patients with breast cancer before systemic therapy: is there an interaction between cancer and comorbidity? J Clin Oncol 2014;32(18):1909–18.
62. Evered L, Scott DA, Silbert B, et al. Postoperative cognitive dysfunction is independent of type of surgery and anesthetic. Anesth Analg 2011;112(5):1179–85.

63. Ewertz M, Jensen AB. Late effects of breast cancer treatment and potentials for rehabilitation. Acta Oncol 2011;50(2):187–93.
64. Runowicz CD, Leach CR, Henry NL, et al. American Cancer Society/American Society of clinical oncology breast cancer survivorship care guideline. J Clin Oncol 2016;34(6):611–35. Available at: http://ascopubs.org/doi/full/10.1200/jco.2015.64.3809.
65. Pullens MJ, De Vries J, Roukema JA. Subjective cognitive dysfunction in breast cancer patients: a systematic review. Psychooncology 2010;19(11):1127–38.
66. O'Farrell E, Smith A, Collins B. Objective-subjective disparity in cancer-related cognitive impairment: does the use of change measures help reconcile the difference? Psychooncology 2016. [Epub ahead of print].
67. Hutchinson A, Hosting J, Kichenadasse G, et al. Objective and subjective cognitive impairment following chemotherapy for cancer: A systematic review. Cancer Treat Rev 2012;38(7):926–34.
68. Ganz PA, Kwan L, Castellon SA, et al. Cognitive complaints after breast cancer treatments: examining the relationship with neuropsychological test performance. J Natl Cancer Inst 2013;105(11):791–801.
69. Meadows AT, Gordon J, Massari DJ, et al. Declines in IQ scores and cognitive dysfunctions in children with acute lymphocytic leukaemia treated with cranial irradiation. Lancet 1981;2(8254):1015–8.
70. Hudson MM, Ness KK, Gurney JG, et al. Clinical ascertainment of health outcomes among adults treated for childhood cancer. JAMA 2013;309(22):2371–81.
71. Krull KR, Brinkman TM, Li C, et al. Neurocognitive outcomes decades after treatment for childhood acute lymphoblastic leukemia: a report from the St Jude lifetime cohort study. J Clin Oncol 2013;31(35):4407–15.
72. Kadan-Lottick NS, Zeltzer LK, Liu Q, et al. Neurocognitive functioning in adult survivors of childhood non-central nervous system cancers. J Natl Cancer Inst 2010; 102(12):881–93.
73. Prasad PK, Hardy KK, Zhang N, et al. Psychosocial and neurocognitive outcomes in adult survivors of adolescent and early young adult cancer: a report from the childhood cancer survivor study. J Clin Oncol 2015;33(23):2545–52.
74. Loh KP, Janelsins MC, Mohile SG, et al. Chemotherapy-related cognitive impairment in older patients with cancer. J Geriatr Oncol 2016;7(4):270–80.
75. Raji MA, Kuo YF, Freeman JL, et al. Effect of a dementia diagnosis on survival of older patients after a diagnosis of breast, colon, or prostate cancer: implications for cancer care. Arch Intern Med 2008;168(18):2033–40.
76. Libert Y, Dubruille S, Borghgraef C, et al. Vulnerabilities in older patients when cancer treatment is initiated: does a cognitive impairment impact the two-year survival? PLoS One 2016;11(8):e0159734.
77. Nasreddine Z, Phillips N, Bedirian V, et al. The montreal cognitive assessment, MoCA: a brief screening tool for mild cognitive impairment. J Am Geriatr Soc 2005;53(4):695–9.
78. Folstein MF, Folstein SE, McHugh PR. "Mini-mental state". A practical method for grading the cognitive state of patients for the clinician. J Psychiatr Res 1975; 12(3):189–98.
79. Wagner LI, Sweet J, Butt Z, et al. Measuring patient self-reported cognitive function: development of the Functional Assessment of Cancer Therapy–Cognitive Function instrument. J Support Oncol 2009;7:W32–9.
80. Wefel JS, Vardy J, Ahles T, et al. International Cognition and Cancer Task Force recommendations to harmonise studies of cognitive function in patients with cancer. Lancet Oncol 2011;12:703–8.

81. Schagen SB, Das E, Vermeulen I. Information about chemotherapy-associated cognitive problems contributes to cognitive problems in cancer patients. Psychooncology 2012;21(10):1132–5.

82. Von Ah D, Storey S, Jansen CE, et al. Coping strategies and interventions for cognitive changes in patients with cancer. Semin Oncol Nurs 2013;29(4):288–99.

83. Cicerone KD, Langenbahn DM, Braden C, et al. Evidence-based cognitive rehabilitation: updated review of the literature from 2003 through 2008. Arch Phys Med Rehabil 2011;92(4):519–30.

84. Ferguson RJ, McDonald BC, Rocque MA, et al. Development of CBT for chemotherapy-related cognitive change: results of a waitlist control trial. Psychooncology 2012;21(2):176–86.

85. Alvarez J, Meyer FL, Granoff DL, et al. The effect of EEG biofeedback on reducing postcancer cognitive impairment. Integr Cancer Ther 2013;12(6): 475–87.

86. Barton DL, Burger K, Novotny PJ, et al. The use of Ginkgo biloba for the prevention of chemotherapy-related cognitive dysfunction in women receiving adjuvant treatment for breast cancer, N00C9. Support Care Cancer 2013;21(4):1185–92.

87. Helal G, Aleisa A, Helal O, et al. Metallothionein induction reduces caspase-3 activity and TNFalpha levels with preservation of cognitive function and intact hippocampal neurons in carmustine-treated rats. Oxid Med Cell Longev 2009;2: 26–35.

88. Lyons L, ELBeltagy M, Bennett G, et al. Fluoxetine counteracts the cognitive and cellular effects of 5-fl uorouracil in the rat hippocampus by a mechanism of prevention rather than recovery. PLoS One 2012;7(1):e30010.

Hormonal Changes and Sexual Dysfunction

Eric S. Zhou, PhD[a,b], Natasha N. Frederick, MD, MPH[b,c], Sharon L. Bober, PhD[a,d,e],*

KEYWORDS

- Sexual dysfunction • Hormone changes • Cancer survivorship
- Cancer treatment side effects

KEY POINTS

- Sexual health is integral to the overall well-being of a patient with cancer and is often impacted by cancer treatment.
- Cancer treatment may interrupt, suppress, or permanently deplete hormonal function in both men and women.
- Physical and psychological interventions are available and can improve sexual health, and/or assist with coping with the dysfunction that results from hormonal changes.
- Patients are interested in receiving further information about their sexual health, but there are barriers that can reduce the likelihood that they will have this conversation with their oncology team.
- Well-designed intervention trials are needed to better understand the impact of systematic approaches to helping patients manage sexual dysfunction.

SEXUALITY AND CANCER

Most patients newly diagnosed with cancer are now likely to survive their disease.[1] With patients with cancer living longer lives following treatment, there is a clear need to address common survivorship challenges faced by the estimated 15 million cancer survivors currently living in the United States.[2] In particular, a survivor's sexuality is a fundamental, life-affirming experience that can be profoundly affected by cancer treatment. There are increasing efforts to understand the complex matter of

The authors have nothing to disclose.
[a] Pediatric Oncology, Perini Family Survivors' Center, Dana-Farber Cancer Institute, 450 Brookline Avenue, Boston, MA 02215, USA; [b] Pediatrics, Harvard Medical School, 25 Shattuck Street, Boston, MA 02115, USA; [c] Pediatric Oncology, Dana-Farber Cancer Institute, 450 Brookline Avenue, Boston, MA 02215, USA; [d] Sexual Health Program, Dana-Farber Cancer Institute, 450 Brookline Avenue, Boston, MA 02215, USA; [e] Psychiatry, Harvard Medical School, 25 Shattuck Street, Boston, MA 02115, USA
* Corresponding author. Sexual Health Program, Dana-Farber Cancer Institute, 450 Brookline Avenue, Boston, MA 02215.
E-mail address: sharon_bober@dfci.harvard.edu

human sexuality from an integrative perspective, rather than focusing solely on physical function and disruptions to organ function.

A number of recent models have been proposed to understand sexual health in the context of cancer care. The Neo-theoretical Framework of Sexuality describes key factors, including sexual self-concept (concerns relevant to body image), sexual relationships (concerns relevant to communication and intimacy), and sexual functioning (concerns relevant to desire, arousal, and excitement).[3] Others have proposed an Integrative Biopsychosocial Model for Intervention, suggesting that a broad approach is necessary to capture the psychological (eg, emotional responses to cancer, body perception, and motivation), interpersonal (eg, changes to couple dynamics, fear of intimacy, and communication barriers), biological (eg, hormonal alterations, body changes, pain, and fatigue), and cultural (eg, religious beliefs, and sexual values and norms) elements that comprise a patient's experience of sexuality.[4] Consistent across these models is the importance that clinicians recognize that sexuality must be seen as more than simply a mechanical event, with proper intervention often requiring a multidisciplinary approach that addresses the multiple facets that can affect sexual health.

TREATMENT-RELATED SEXUAL DYSFUNCTION AND HORMONAL THERAPY

Providers should avoid making the assumption that all patients with cancer will present with the same types of sexual dysfunction, even if they have the same diagnoses and treatments. Generally speaking, estimates of the prevalence of sexual dysfunction after cancer range from 40% to 100%, affecting both sexes.[5–7] It is broadly acknowledged that all major treatment modalities have potential to significantly disrupt male and female sexual function.[8] Common treatment-related side effects include disorders of sexual response, desire, and motivation. Both men and women may experience difficulty with arousal, orgasmic dysfunction, hypoactive sexual desire, body image disturbances, and lowered sexual self-esteem. Men may experience erectile dysfunction, and ejaculatory dysfunction. Women may suffer from reduced lubrication, and chronic dyspareunia.[9] Please refer to **Table 1** for a summary of possible sexual health consequences of cancer treatment.

Hormonal therapies that interrupt, suppress, or permanently deplete hormonal function have profound impact on sexual function.[10] However, distressing sexual problems related to hormonal therapy are not consistently identified by clinicians and may be overlooked entirely.[11,12] This is of particular significance because both frequency and duration of use of hormonal therapies with both male and female patients is steadily increasing.[13,14] The following sections overview common issues around sexual dysfunction related to hormonal therapy for men and women. We also make note of several subpopulations of patients who experience significant treatment-related sexual dysfunction related to hormonal interruption/dysfunction that are often overlooked.

Breast Cancer

Treatment for breast cancer can involve a combination of surgery, chemotherapy, radiation therapy, and/or hormone therapy. Women's sexual health is potentially impacted by all of these treatments,[15,16] and distressing sexual concerns commonly affect 30% to 100% of survivors.[17] The negative sexual side effects of chemotherapy treatment that depletes circulating reproductive hormones are well described in the literature[18] and have been shown to be particularly distressing for women.[19–22] More specifically, chemotherapy-related hypoestrogenism results in multiple effects on the vagina and vulva.[23] The epithelium thins, loses cornification and rugation, and blood flow is decreased; causing tissue to become smooth, pale, and fragile. Vaginal secretions are decreased and pH increases. There is a loss of collagen, hyalinization, and elastin, and the vagina may narrow or shorten. This vulvovaginal atrophy is often accompanied by decreased libido and adverse effects on sexual arousal and orgasm.[24] For young women with breast cancer, ovarian failure induced by chemotherapy may be associated with a more comprehensive loss of ovarian function than in natural menopause.[25] Chemotherapy results in premature ovarian failure in 30% to 96% of premenopausal women,[26] with the highest risk for women older than 40 years (50%–96%) and those exposed to alkylating agents such as cyclophosphamide.[27] Beyond these common physical side effects of estrogen-deprivation, women who undergo hormonal disruption also report distress around decreased sense of intimacy, and diminished partner function.[15,28–30] Loss of sexual function and satisfaction with intimacy have been associated with poorer quality of life for breast cancer survivors.[31]

There is now a steadily increasing use of endocrine therapies with both older and younger patients with breast cancer and survivors.[10,13] Endocrine therapies typically also result in a raft of menopausal symptoms that patients are often not prepared to manage.[25] For more than 2 decades, 5 years or more of adjuvant tamoxifen has been the standard of care for premenopausal breast cancer survivors.[32] Large-scale studies have generally not found sexual dysfunction to be a common treatment-related side effect of this endocrine treatment.[33] However, the American Society of Clinical Oncology has revised clinical practice guidelines and now recommends the use of adjuvant ovarian suppression therapy with young female survivors of estrogen-positive breast cancer.[34] This means there is an increasing use of treatments to suppress ovarian function in young, premenopausal women and recent evidence regarding treatment-related sexual dysfunction is striking.[35] Marked vulvovaginal atrophy, loss of arousal and desire, and loss of sexual satisfaction are common, and sexual problems related to ovarian suppression do not resolve over time.[36]

Table 1
Cancer-directed treatment side effects that can impact sexual function

Sexual Dysfunction		
Male	**Female**	**Male and Female**
Erectile dysfunction	Dyspareunia	Reduced libido
Dry/painful orgasm	Vaginal atrophy	Pain
Ejaculatory dysfunction	Loss of nipple sensation	Chronic fatigue
		Nausea/vomiting
		Lymphedema
		Urinary incontinence
		Bowel incontinence
		Scars
		Amputations
		Ostomies
		Problems with arousal
		Reduced sexual motivation
		Decreased body image
		Loss of sexual self-esteem

For postmenopausal survivors, aromatase inhibitors remain the preferred first line of adjuvant endocrine therapy to reduce risk of cancer recurrence.[34] Aromatase inhibitors act as estrogen antagonists in the vagina,[37] which often leads to severe dyspareunia.[20] In systematic review of prospective data from randomized trials and an observational study comparing aromatase inhibitors with tamoxifen, the prevalence and severity of vaginal dryness and dyspareunia are worse with aromatase inhibitors than with tamoxifen.[38] In addition to the intense menopause-related symptoms of vulvovaginal atrophy,[39] women on aromatase inhibitors are at significantly increased risk for lichen sclerosus, a perineal skin condition that results in itching, burning, and thin, crinkled skin prone to bruising and tearing.[40] If untreated, this condition can lead to scarring, ulcerations, and labial fusion, all of which make sexual activity painful and potentially unattainable.[41] Lichen sclerosus also raises risk for vulvar cancer. Given the potential risk of lichen sclerosus in women who are severely estrogen-depleted, it has been proposed that all women on an aromatase-inhibitor undergo yearly vulvovaginal examinations to rule out lichen sclerosus and other vulvovaginal side effects of treatment.[40]

Prostate Cancer

Men on hormone therapy similarly experience pronounced sexual side effects. The primary treatment for men diagnosed with late-stage prostate cancer is hormone therapy, also referred to as androgen deprivation therapy (ADT). Broader use of ADT in men has been increasing, with ADT now being used regularly for men diagnosed with localized high-risk disease.[42–44] The purpose of hormone therapy for men is to reduce the level of androgens to minimize their potential impact on the progression of prostate cancer cells. Men on ADT are essentially chemically castrated to manage aggressive prostate disease. When testosterone is depleted, nitric oxide levels drop and there is loss of intracavernosal pressure, which results in erectile dysfunction. In addition to erectile dysfunction, side effects of ADT also include body feminization, profound loss of libido, hot flashes, and emotional lability.[45–47] The severe hormone-related side effects are equally similar in men who are treated for either localized[44,48] or metastatic disease.[49–52] Today in North America, there are more than half a million men on ADT and most men are on ADT for several years.[53] The extreme sexual and quality-of-life side effects of ADT also negatively impact partners. It has been shown that both patients and partners feel unprepared to manage these problems.[54]

Testicular Cancer

Testicular cancer is typically treated with surgery, and potentially followed with radiation therapy or chemotherapy.[55–57] Sexual problems are reported by 12% to 40% of testicular cancer survivors regardless of type of treatment[58] and they include difficulties with sexual desire, ejaculatory difficulties, and erectile dysfunction.[59–62] Testicular cancer survivors also may be self-conscious about changes in physical/testicular appearance and a perceived loss of masculinity. Although treatment-related sexual problems are not always organic, rates of subnormal levels of testosterone range from approximately 10% to 15% in testicular cancer survivors.[63] As a result, testicular cancer survivors with decreased hormonal function often report reductions in sexual activity levels and general sexual dissatisfaction following treatment.[64,65] Thus, it is important for clinicians to also assess hormonal function in testicular cancer survivors who report having bothersome sexual problems.

Impact of Risk-Reducing Surgery: BRCA Mutation Carriers

Women who are BRCA1/2 carriers face a high lifetime risk for breast (55%–85%) and/ or ovarian cancer (15%–44%).[66] For these women, risk-reducing salpingo-oophorectomy (RRSO) is recommended by age 35 or after completion of child-bearing. RRSO reduces risk of ovarian cancer by more than 80% and also lowers breast cancer risk by half.[67] This preventive risk-reducing surgery successfully reduces cancer risk, but also can lead to a range of sexual side effects that are highly distressing. Comparable to those side effects previously discussed in the section describing ovarian suppression, women who undergo RRSO similarly are at risk for vaginal dryness, vulvovaginal atrophy, and loss of arousal and genital sensation.[68] The most frequently cited postsurgical concerns of mutation carriers are the sexual side effects, and women express that they wished they had received counseling about this topic.[69]

Stem Cell Transplantation

Long-term posttransplant complications can cause significant quality-of-life impairments for those who underwent stem cell transplantation (SCT).[70] Endocrine disruptions can be caused by chemotherapy, radiation therapy, and SCT, with many issues the result of conditioning regimens with total body irradiation and/or chemotherapy.[71] Consequently, late-effects guidelines recommend that patients who have undergone SCT receive annual screenings for endocrine function (eg, thyroid function).[70] Gonadal dysfunction is commonly seen in SCT recipients, with reported rates as high as 92% for male and 99% for female patients.[72–74] Although rates of gonadal dysfunction will vary depending on individual variables (eg, age, conditioning regimen), women are generally more likely to experience problems than men. Notably, ovarian endocrine failure in adult women is usually irreversible,[75,76] although there is recent evidence to suggest that reduced-intensity condition regimens may protect ovarian function.[77] Women who experience ovarian failure are likely to suffer from significant sexual health consequences, including poorer body image (the result of hypertrichosis and Cushing syndrome, for example), lowered libido, and vaginal dryness. Consequently, women who undergo SCT report a greater decrement in frequency of sexual relations than men.[78] Men also experience sexual difficulties following SCT. Approximately 10% report difficulty with erectile function and/or ejaculation, and the conditioning regimen can cause testicular damage in men with low testosterone levels.[78,79] Women are encouraged to discuss the potential use of hormonal replacement therapy and vaginal lubrication, and both men and women should be openly discussing sexual health with their medical providers before transplantation has occurred.[70,78]

Adolescent and Young Adult Cancer

Medical advances in pediatric oncology now ensure that more than 80% of children and adolescents diagnosed with cancer will survive.[80] Research shows that disruption of psychosexual development and sexual dysfunction are profoundly distressing long-term side effects of pediatric cancer treatment.[81,82] Almost half of young adult survivors of childhood cancer struggle with at least 1 major sexual problem,[12,83] and 30% report 2 or more problems.[12] Such problems include pain, difficulty with orgasm, lack of desire, and arousal difficulties. Additionally, research focusing on patients treated between the ages of 15 and 39 years found that 49% of Adolescent and young adult (AYA) reported negative effects on sexual function 1 year after cancer diagnosis and 70% of those persisted with negative perceptions at 2 years after diagnosis.[84] These stand in contrast to reports of sexual dysfunction in the general adolescent and young adult population, where rates fall between 10% and 15% for women and men, respectively.[85] The age at which a child is diagnosed with cancer can be important with respect to their later life sexual health. For example, girls who received SCT before puberty are more likely to avoid ovarian failure, and subsequent sexual side effects, that is far more common in adults who undergo SCT. These younger patients often require sex hormone replacement therapy post-SCT.[86] Similarly, girls who undergo SCT at a younger age (<13 years) are more likely to maintain fertility. In contrast, boys who underwent SCT before puberty were at greater risk for infertility.[87]

Research focused on adult cancer survivors shows clear relationships between cancer treatments, such as chemotherapy, and hormonal therapy, with direct damage to sexual organs and/or hormonal systems resulting in sexual dysfunction.[24,88–92] In contrast, studies in childhood cancer survivors have shown that in addition to disruptions in endocrine function among other physical late effects, psychosocial factors, such as anxiety, fear of partner rejection, fear of being pitied, and poor self-esteem, also play a significant role in the development of sexual problems.[11,12,83] For example, negative body image can develop secondary to the physical changes incurred by cancer treatment and plays a prominent role in social and sexual interactions during treatment, potentially contributing to delayed physical and emotional intimacy, and continues well into survivorship.[84,93] Given that negative body image in adolescence can impede the development of a healthy sexual identity,[94] and that body image issues often remain after active treatment, it is critical for clinicians to routinely address body image concerns in addition to acknowledging and assessing changes in hormonal function.

MANAGING SEXUAL DYSFUNCTION
Evaluation

Effective interventions can be delivered only if an adequate assessment about the patient's sexuality has occurred. The use of screening tools can be helpful as a brief, preliminary approach to assessing sexual function in cancer survivors, and to determine which patients may benefit from further discussion about their symptoms. The use of screening instruments can help with starting conversations with patients and their families.

In women, the Female Sexual Function Index (FSFI) is a measure of sexual function that has been validated in female cancer populations.[95] This is a 19-item self-report measure that assesses function "over the past 4 weeks" in the following specific domains relevant to female sexuality: desire, arousal, lubrication, orgasm, satisfaction, and pain.[96] The FSFI has been used in research conducted with patients with cancer and survivor studies,[97,98] and is able to differentiate between clinical and nonclinical populations.[95] The scale, along with instructions for use and scoring, are available at www.FSFIquestionnaire.com.[95] For providers who are working with men, the International Index of Erectile Function (IIEF) can be a valuable tool.[99] The IIEF is a 15-item self-report measure that is available in multiple languages.[99] It has been used in studies with patients with prostate cancer[97] and asks about sexual function "over the past 4 weeks." The IIEF asks about the following domains relevant to male sexuality: erectile function, orgasm, desire, intercourse satisfaction, and overall satisfaction.

The use of screening measures should be designed to help facilitate a subsequent conversation, instead of as a replacement of a full clinical assessment. This discussion can be guided by a structured model of clinical inquiry. An example of a popular model is the BETTER model.[100] The model's name stands for *Bringing up the topic of sexual* health during consults, *E*xplain to the patient that sexuality is a part of cancer care, *T*ell the patient that resources are available to address sexual health, *T*ime discussions and emphasize that patients can bring the topic up at any time, *E*ducate the patient about the possible changes in sexuality that can result from cancer treatment, and *R*ecord the discussion in the patient's chart. Alternatively, the PLISSIT Model offers another framework to consider.[101] PLISSIT stands for asking *P*ermission to talk about sexuality, offering *L*imited *I*nformation to address sexual concerns, providing *S*pecific *S*uggestions based on the patient's presentation, and referring for *I*ntensive *T*herapy as indicated based on symptom report.

Intervention

Without intervention, the negative impact of sexual dysfunction on patients with cancer is significant and evidence suggests that these problems often get worse over time.[102,103] An overarching model that can guide a provider in appreciating the intervention process is the Five A's Framework, which focuses on 5 important facets of treatment: Ask, Advise, Assess, Assist, and Arrange.[104] In this model, the provider makes sure that all cancer survivors are *Asked* about their sexual health using a nonjudgmental approach. Next, the provider must demonstrate willingness to *Advise* the survivor that his or her problems are normative and that treatment options exist. Third, a provider must adequately *Assess* the survivor's sexual dysfunction. Subsequently, the patient can be *Assisted* through specific therapeutic efforts, ranging from psychoeducation, to referrals, to active treatment. Finally, a provider must ensure that he or she *Arranges* follow-up so that the patient's status is routinely monitored.

It is important that a clinician who treats cancer survivors develops a multidisciplinary network of referrals to address sexual concerns from an integrative perspective. Individuals on this list are likely to include the following:

- Urologist
- Gynecologist
- Endocrinologist
- Cardiologist
- Primary care physician
- Pelvic floor physical therapist
- Psychologist

Women

As described, one of the most commonly reported post–cancer treatment symptoms for women is vaginal dryness. This can be debilitating for women because of physical consequences, such as pain, chafing, and bleeding, all of which can subsequently lead to significant reductions in sexual desire. First-line treatment includes vaginal lubricants and moisturizers. Vaginal lubricants provide topical lubrication and promote comfort during sexual activity, and, if used properly, can help to prevent irritation and potentially avoid mucosal tears. Unlike lubricants, vaginal moisturizers are intended to be used consistently for overall vaginal comfort and are not used on an as-needed basis during sexual activity. Moisturizers are designed to hydrate the vaginal mucosa and should be used routinely by cancer survivors who experience regular vaginal dryness. Rather than focusing on the particular formula used for an individual vaginal moisturizer, evidence indicates that the benefit of vaginal moisturizers depends on consistent use up to 5 times per week. Further, female cancer survivors can consider the use of vaginal dilator therapy, especially if they have received pelvic radiation. Dilator therapy helps to maintain vaginal length and caliber after radiation therapy by preventing adherence of the vaginal walls, and long-term use after pelvic radiation therapy may be important to prevent fibrosis and ensure overall vaginal health.[105,106] In addition, exercises designed to tense and relax the muscles around the vaginal introitus can improve pelvic muscle floor strength and tone and vaginal elasticity, which have been associated with reductions in vaginal pain[107,108] and better sexual functioning.[109]

Men

Addressing the sexual health symptoms that are commonly reported by male cancer survivors may involve collaboration with medical specialists, such as urologists who treat male sexual dysfunction. The most common challenge that a male cancer survivor will report to providers is erectile dysfunction. To treat erectile dysfunction, oral phosphodiesterase type 5 (PDE-5) inhibitors are often used at the initial therapy, as they are effective and minimally invasive.[110] It is noted that discontinuation of PDE-5 inhibitors can occur due to both physical (eg, headache, muscle pain, dyspepsia, facial flushing) and psychological issues (eg, anxiety about medication use, having to plan/schedule romantic activity).[111,112] Moreover, PDE-5 inhibitors may not be effective when men have nerve or vascular damage; for example, when there is trauma or permanent damage to nerves after radical prostatectomy, Alternatives to oral PDE-5 inhibitors include intracavernous injection therapy, transurethral alprostadil, and vacuum erection devices, all of which can be very effective for these men.[113–115] Specific to men who have undergone hormonal therapy, decrements to their libido are a common concern that also must be addressed. This is a difficult issue to treat, as medical options (eg, increasing testosterone levels) directly oppose the efforts at cancer therapy. There are behavioral and psychological interventions designed to facilitate improved couple's communication, reduce relationship distress, identify novel nonpenetrative intercourse sexually stimulating activities, and improve coping skills that can be helpful for the patient and his partner.[116–121]

Relationship function

Physical sexual dysfunction due to cancer treatment can often be the precipitant that causes partners to reevaluate other issues in that particular relationship. For example, it is possible that the cancer survivor and his or her partner are facing general relationship distress,[122,123] or struggling with poor overall communication[124] instead of a specific sexual side effect. Incorporating the "cancer dyad" into any discussion that involves sexual functioning could be crucial to the success of an intervention effort.[125] Evidence suggests that having both partners present is helpful for both individuals during the cancer recovery process.[126,127]

Challenges

Despite the awareness that sexual function is often affected significantly by cancer treatment and subsequent hormonal disruptions, most cancer survivors are not adequately evaluated and treated for their symptoms. Patients with cancer want information about how they can cope with sexual health changes,[128] but find themselves disappointed by the lack of information, support, and practical strategies provided by their clinicians to help manage the sexual changes secondary to cancer and cancer treatments.[129–131] By not adequately discussing sexual health during routine medical visits, clinicians may be mistakenly providing patients with the message that their sexual dysfunction cannot be adequately treated. The discomfort that medical providers experience when addressing sexual problems[132] appears to fall into 3 categories: issues related to patient characteristics, provider characteristics, and systems issues.[104] The patient characteristics describe the provider's assumptions about their patient's sexuality due to individual characteristics, such as age, gender, partner status, sexual orientation, prognosis, and socioeconomic status. Next, the provider characteristics refer to the training, experience, knowledge, and attitudes of that particular provider, with a lack of experience and knowledge often reported as the reason for why sexuality is not sufficiently addressed during routine cancer care.[133,134] Finally, systems issues include problems such as insufficient time during medical appointments to discuss sexual health, in the context of the multitude of other survivorship concerns.[133]

SUMMARY

Now that most cancer survivors are living many years beyond diagnosis and treatment, it is imperative for medical providers to discuss a patient's sexual heath after cancer treatment. Acknowledging the general lack of formal training in sexual medicine, it is important that clinicians seek out support so that they can feel comfortable in addressing this common concern for patients during survivorship. For this reason, we strongly advise providers to build a referral list of either hospital-based or community-based colleagues who can help comanage these issues. We also encourage providers to maintain an awareness of sexual dysfunction in the context of seeing survivors who do not necessarily present with more obvious comorbid side effects of treatment, such as fatigue or physical pain. This is likely most readily achieved by assessing sexual function as part of a general and routine review of systems. As patients struggle to regain quality of life and a sense of healing after cancer, simply inquiring about sexual problems both acknowledges and validates an experience that is often taboo, Finally, it is reassuring that for many cancer survivors, even a limited amount of education helping the patient understand basic treatment options (eg, vaginal lubricants and moisturizers for women, and oral PDE-5 inhibitors for men) can be very helpful. Given that most cancer patients and survivors do not receive treatment targeted to this underaddressed facet of their health, it is not only helpful but also empowering for survivors when they can gain significant improvements in quality of life from specific strategies aimed at ameliorating treatment-related sexual problems.

REFERENCES

1. Howlader N, Noone AM, Krapcho M, et al. SEER Cancer Statistics Review, 1975-2010. Bethesda (MD): National Cancer Institute; 2013. Based on November 2012 SEER data submission, posted to the SEER Web site.

2. DeSantis CE, Lin CC, Mariotto AB, et al. Cancer treatment and survivorship statistics, 2014. CA Cancer J Clin 2014;64(4):252–71.

3. Cleary V, Hegarty J. Understanding sexuality in women with gynaecological cancer. Eur J Oncol Nurs 2011;15(1):38–45.

4. Bober SL, Varela VS. Sexuality in adult cancer survivors: challenges and intervention. J Clin Oncol 2012;30(30):3712–9.

5. Derogatis LR, Kourlesis SM. An approach to evaluation of sexual problems in the cancer patient. CA Cancer J Clin 1981;31(1):46–50.

6. Ganz PA, Rowland JH, Desmond K, et al. Life after breast cancer: understanding women's health-related quality of life and sexual functioning. J Clin Oncol 1998;16(2):501–14.

7. Stanford JL, Feng Z, Hamilton AS, et al. Urinary and sexual function after radical prostatectomy for clinically localized prostate cancer: the Prostate Cancer Outcomes Study. JAMA 2000;283(3):354–60.

8. Schover LR. Counseling cancer patients about changes in sexual function. Oncology (Williston Park) 1999;13(11):1585–91 [discussion: 1591–2, 1595–6].

9. Basson R, Schultz WW. Sexual sequelae of general medical disorders. Lancet 2007;369(9559):409–24.

10. Jain S, Santa-Maria CA, Gradishar WJ. The role of ovarian suppression in premenopausal women with hormone receptor-positive early-stage breast cancer. Oncology 2015;29(7):473.

11. Frederick NN, Recklitis CJ, Blackmon JE, et al. Sexual dysfunction in young adult survivors of childhood cancer. Pediatr Blood Cancer 2016;63(9):1622–8.

12. Bober SL, Zhou ES, Chen B, et al. Sexual function in childhood cancer survivors: a report from Project REACH. J Sex Med 2013;10(8):2084–93.

13. Goss PE, Ingle JN, Pritchard KI, et al. Extending aromatase-inhibitor adjuvant therapy to 10 years. N Engl J Med 2016;375(3):209–19.

14. Pether M, Goldenberg S, Bhagirath K, et al. Intermittent androgen suppression in prostate cancer: an update of the Vancouver experience. Can J Urol 2003; 10(2):1809–14.

15. Katz A. Breast cancer and women's sexuality. Am J Nurs 2011;111(4):63–7.

16. Bredart A, Dolbeault S, Savignoni A, et al. Prevalence and associated factors of sexual problems after early-stage breast cancer treatment: results of a French exploratory survey. Psychooncology 2011;20(8):841–50.

17. Sadovsky R, Basson R, Krychman M, et al. Cancer and sexual problems. J Sex Med 2010;7(1 Pt 2):349–73.

18. Goldfarb S, Mulhall J, Nelson C, et al. Sexual and reproductive health in cancer survivors. Semin Oncol 2013;40(6):726–44.

19. Baumgart J, Nilsson K, Stavreus-Evers A, et al. Urogenital disorders in women with adjuvant endocrine therapy after early breast cancer. Am J Obstet Gynecol 2011;204(1):26.e1–7.

20. Baumgart J, Nilsson K, Evers AS, et al. Sexual dysfunction in women on adjuvant endocrine therapy after breast cancer. Menopause 2013;20(2):162–8.

21. Gallicchio L, MacDonald R, Wood B, et al. Menopausal-type symptoms among breast cancer patients on aromatase inhibitor therapy. Climacteric 2012;15(4): 339–49.

22. Safarinejad MR, Shafiei N, Safarinejad S. Quality of life and sexual functioning in young women with early-stage breast cancer 1 year after lumpectomy. Psychooncology 2013;22(6):1242–8.

23. Lev-Sagie A. Vulvar and vaginal atrophy: physiology, clinical presentation, and treatment considerations. Clin Obstet Gynecol 2015;58(3):476–91.

24. Schover LR. Premature ovarian failure and its consequences: vasomotor symptoms, sexuality, and fertility. J Clin Oncol 2008;26(5):753–8.

25. Shuster LT, Rhodes DJ, Gostout BS, et al. Premature menopause or early menopause: long-term health consequences. Maturitas 2010;65(2):161–6.

26. Rosenberg SM, Partridge AH. Premature menopause in young breast cancer: effects on quality of life and treatment interventions. J Thorac Dis 2013; 5(Suppl 1):S55–61.

27. Anchan RM, Ginsburg ES. Fertility concerns and preservation in younger women with breast cancer. Crit Rev Oncol Hematol 2010;74(3):175–92.

28. Dizon DS. Quality of life after breast cancer: survivorship and sexuality. Breast J 2009;15(5):500–4.

29. Emilee G, Ussher JM, Perz J. Sexuality after breast cancer: a review. Maturitas 2010;66(4):397–407.
30. Elmir R, Jackson D, Beale B, et al. Against all odds: Australian women's experiences of recovery from breast cancer. J Clin Nurs 2010;19(17–18):2531–8.
31. Reese JB, Shelby RA, Keefe FJ, et al. Sexual concerns in cancer patients: a comparison of GI and breast cancer patients. Support Care Cancer 2010; 18(9):1179–89.
32. National Comprehensive Cancer Network. NCCN clinical practice guidelines in oncology: breast cancer. Version 3.2014. Available at: https://www.nccn.org/professionals/physician_gls/pdf/breast.pdf.
33. Tevaarwerk AJ, Wang M, Zhao F, et al. Phase III comparison of tamoxifen versus tamoxifen plus ovarian function suppression in premenopausal women with node-negative, hormone receptor–positive breast cancer (E-3193, INT-0142): a trial of the Eastern Cooperative Oncology Group. J Clin Oncol 2014;32(35): 3948–58.
34. Rugo HS, Rumble RB, Macrae E, et al. Endocrine therapy for hormone receptor–positive metastatic breast cancer: American Society of Clinical Oncology Guideline. J Clin Oncol 2016;34(25):3069–103.
35. Ribi K, Luo W, Bernhard J, et al. Adjuvant tamoxifen plus ovarian function suppression versus tamoxifen alone in premenopausal women with early breast cancer: patient-reported outcomes in the suppression of ovarian function Trial. J Clin Oncol 2016;34(14):1601–10.
36. Frechette D, Paquet L, Verma S, et al. The impact of endocrine therapy on sexual dysfunction in postmenopausal women with early stage breast cancer: encouraging results from a prospective study. Breast Cancer Res Treat 2013; 141(1):111–7.
37. Mortimer JE, Boucher L, Baty J, et al. Effect of tamoxifen on sexual functioning in patients with breast cancer. J Clin Oncol 1999;17(5):1488–92.
38. Mok K, Juraskova I, Friedlander M. The impact of aromatase inhibitors on sexual functioning: current knowledge and future research directions. Breast 2008; 17(5):436–40.
39. Cella D, Fallowfield L, Barker P, et al. Quality of life of postmenopausal women in the ATAC ("Arimidex", tamoxifen, alone or in combination) trial after completion of 5 years' adjuvant treatment for early breast cancer. Breast Cancer Res Treat 2006;100(3):273–84.
40. Potter JE, Moore KA. Lichen sclerosus in a breast cancer survivor on an aromatase inhibitor: a case report. J Gen Intern Med 2013;28(4):592–5.
41. Funaro D. Lichen sclerosus: a review and practical approach. Dermatol Ther 2004;17(1):28–37.
42. Heidenreich A, Bellmunt J, Bolla M, et al. EAU guidelines on prostate cancer. Part I: screening, diagnosis, and treatment of clinically localised disease. Actas Urol Esp 2011;35(9):501–14 [in Spanish].
43. Mottet N, Bellmunt J, Bolla M, et al. EAU guidelines on prostate cancer. Part II: treatment of advanced, relapsing, and castration-resistant prostate cancer. Actas Urol Esp 2011;35(10):565–79 [in Spanish].
44. Potosky AL, Reeve BB, Clegg LX, et al. Quality of life following localized prostate cancer treated initially with androgen deprivation therapy or no therapy. J Natl Cancer Inst 2002;94(6):430–7.
45. Alibhai SM, Gogov S, Allibhai Z. Long-term side effects of androgen deprivation therapy in men with non-metastatic prostate cancer: a systematic literature review. Crit Rev Oncol Hematol 2006;60(3):201–15.

46. Holzbeierlein JM, McLaughlin MD, Thrasher JB. Complications of androgen deprivation therapy for prostate cancer. Curr Opin Urol 2004;14(3):177–83.

47. Elliott S, Latini DM, Walker LM, et al. Androgen deprivation therapy for prostate cancer: recommendations to improve patient and partner quality of life. J Sex Med 2010;7(9):2996–3010.

48. Gacci M, Simonato A, Masieri L, et al. Urinary and sexual outcomes in long-term (5+ years) prostate cancer disease free survivors after radical prostatectomy. Health Qual Life Outcomes 2009;7(1):94.

49. Litwin MS, Shpall AI, Dorey F, et al. Quality-of-life outcomes in long-term survivors of advanced prostate cancer. Am J Clin Oncol 1998;21(4):327–32.

50. Albertsen PC, Aaronson NK, Muller MJ, et al. Health-related quality of life among patients with metastatic prostate cancer. Urology 1997;49(2):207–16 [discussion: 216–7].

51. Herr HW, Kornblith AB, Ofman U. A comparison of the quality of life of patients with metastatic prostate cancer who received or did not receive hormonal therapy. Cancer 1993;71(3 Suppl):1143–50.

52. Herr HW, O'Sullivan M. Quality of life of asymptomatic men with nonmetastatic prostate cancer on androgen deprivation therapy. J Urol 2000;163(6):1743–6.

53. Smith MR. Androgen deprivation therapy for prostate cancer: new concepts and concerns. Curr Opin Endocrinol Diabetes Obes 2007;14(3):247.

54. Walker LM, Robinson JW. A description of heterosexual couples' sexual adjustment to androgen deprivation therapy for prostate cancer. Psychooncology 2011;20(8):880–8.

55. Laguna MP, Pizzocaro G, Klepp O, et al. EAU guidelines on testicular cancer. Eur Urol 2001;40(2):102–10.

56. Albers P, Albrecht W, Algaba F, et al. EAU guidelines on testicular cancer: 2011 update. Eur Urol 2011;60(2):304–19.

57. Albers P, Albrecht W, Algaba F, et al. Guidelines on testicular cancer: 2015 update. Eur Urol 2015;68(6):1054–68.

58. Wiechno P, Demkow T, Kubiak K, et al. The quality of life and hormonal disturbances in testicular cancer survivors in cisplatin era. Eur Urol 2007;52(5):1448–54.

59. Brodsky MS. Testicular cancer survivors' impressions of the impact of the disease on their lives. Qual Health Res 1995;5(1):78–96.

60. Kuczyk M, Machtens S, Bokemeyer C, et al. Sexual function and fertility after treatment of testicular cancer. Curr Opin Urol 2000;10(5):473–7.

61. Dahl AA, Bremnes R, Dahl O, et al. Is the sexual function compromised in long-term testicular cancer survivors? Eur Urol 2007;52(5):1438–47.

62. Jonker-Pool G, Van de Wiel HB, Hoekstra HJ, et al. Sexual functioning after treatment for testicular cancer–review and meta-analysis of 36 empirical studies between 1975-2000. Arch Sex Behav 2001;30(1):55–74.

63. Huddart RA, Norman A, Moynihan C, et al. Fertility, gonadal and sexual function in survivors of testicular cancer. Br J Cancer 2005;93(2):200–7.

64. Rossen P, Pedersen AF, Zachariae R, et al. Sexuality and body image in long-term survivors of testicular cancer. Eur J Cancer 2012;48(4):571–8.

65. Nazareth I, Lewin J, King M. Sexual dysfunction after treatment for testicular cancer: a systematic review. J Psychosom Res 2001;51(6):735–43.

66. King MC, Marks JH, Mandell JB, Group New York Breast Cancer Study. Breast and ovarian cancer risks due to inherited mutations in BRCA1 and BRCA2. Science 2003;302(5645):643–6.

67. Domchek SM, Friebel TM, Singer CF, et al. Association of risk-reducing surgery in BRCA1 or BRCA2 mutation carriers with cancer risk and mortality. JAMA 2010;304(9):967–75.
68. Carter J, Goldfrank D, Schover LR. Simple strategies for vaginal health promotion in cancer survivors. J Sex Med 2011;8(2):549–59.
69. Campfield Bonadies D, Moyer A, Matloff ET. What I wish I'd known before surgery: BRCA carriers' perspectives after bilateral salipingo-oophorectomy. Fam Cancer 2011;10(1):79–85.
70. Majhail NS, Rizzo JD, Lee SJ, et al. Recommended screening and preventive practices for long-term survivors after hematopoietic cell transplantation. Hematol Oncol Stem Cell Ther 2012;5(1):1–30.
71. Brennan BM, Shalet SM. Endocrine late effects after bone marrow transplant. Br J Haematol 2002;118(1):58–66.
72. Mertens A, Ramsay N, Kouris S, et al. Patterns of gonadal dysfunction following bone marrow transplantation. Bone Marrow Transplant 1998;22(4):345–50.
73. Afify Z, Shaw P, Clavano-Harding A, et al. Growth and endocrine function in children with acute myeloid leukaemia after bone marrow transplantation using busulfan/cyclophosphamide. Bone Marrow Transplant 2000;25(10):1087.
74. Ranke M, Schwarze C, Dopfer R, et al. Late effects after stem cell transplantation (SCT) in children–growth and hormones. Bone Marrow Transplant 2005;35: S77–81.
75. Sanders JE. Endocrine complications of high-dose therapy with stem cell transplantation. Pediatr Transplant 2004;8(s5):39–50.
76. Spinelli S, Chiodi S, Bacigalupo A, et al. Ovarian recovery after total body irradiation and allogeneic bone marrow transplantation: long-term follow up of 79 females. Bone Marrow Transplant 1994;14(3):373–80.
77. Phelan R, Mann E, Napurski C, et al. Ovarian function after hematopoietic cell transplantation: a descriptive study following the use of GnRH agonists for myeloablative conditioning and observation only for reduced-intensity conditioning. Bone Marrow Transplant 2016;51(10):1369–75.
78. Chiodi S, Spinelli S, Ravera G, et al. Quality of life in 244 recipients of allogeneic bone marrow transplantation. Br J Haematol 2000;110(3):614–9.
79. Marks D, Crilley P, Nezu C, et al. Sexual dysfunction prior to high-dose chemotherapy and bone marrow transplantation. Bone Marrow Transplant 1996;17(4): 595–9.
80. Mariotto AB, Rowland JH, Yabroff KR, et al. Long-term survivors of childhood cancers in the United States. Cancer Epidemiol Biomarkers Prev 2009;18(4): 1033–40.
81. Schover LR. Sexuality and fertility after cancer. Hematol Am Soc Hematol Educ Program 2005;1:523–7.
82. Schover LR. Patient attitudes toward fertility preservation. Pediatr Blood Cancer 2009;53(2):281–4.
83. Zebrack BJ, Foley S, Wittmann D, et al. Sexual functioning in young adult survivors of childhood cancer. Psychooncology 2010;19(8):814–22.
84. Wettergren L, Kent EE, Mitchell SA, et al. Cancer negatively impacts on sexual function in adolescents and young adults: the Aya Hope study. Psychooncology 2016.
85. Flynn KE, Lindau ST, Lin L, et al. Development and validation of a single-item screener for self-reporting sexual problems in U.S. adults. J Gen Intern Med 2015;30(10):1468–75.

86. Socié G, Salooja N, Cohen A, et al. Nonmalignant late effects after allogeneic stem cell transplantation. Blood 2003;101(9):3373–85.

87. Borgmann-Staudt A, Rendtorff R, Reinmuth S, et al. Fertility after allogeneic haematopoietic stem cell transplantation in childhood and adolescence. Bone Marrow Transplant 2012;47(2):271–6.

88. Ganz PA, Greendale GA, Petersen L, et al. Breast cancer in younger women: reproductive and late health effects of treatment. J Clin Oncol 2003;21(22): 4184–93.

89. Hollenbeck BK, Dunn RL, Wei JT, et al. Sexual health recovery after prostatectomy, external radiation, or brachytherapy for early stage prostate cancer. Curr Urol Rep 2004;5(3):212–9.

90. Potosky AL, Davis WW, Hoffman RM, et al. Five-year outcomes after prostatectomy or radiotherapy for prostate cancer: the prostate cancer outcomes study. J Natl Cancer Inst 2004;96(18):1358–67.

91. Burwell SR, Case LD, Kaelin C, et al. Sexual problems in younger women after breast cancer surgery. J Clin Oncol 2006;24(18):2815–21.

92. Sundberg KK, Lampic C, Arvidson J, et al. Sexual function and experience among long-term survivors of childhood cancer. Eur J Cancer 2011;47(3): 397–403.

93. Wallace ML, Harcourt D, Rumsey N, et al. Managing appearance changes resulting from cancer treatment: resilience in adolescent females. Psychooncology 2007;16(11):1019–27.

94. Evan EE, Kaufman M, Cook AB, et al. Sexual health and self-esteem in adolescents and young adults with cancer. Cancer 2006;107(7 Suppl):1672–9.

95. Rosen R, Brown C, Heiman J, et al. The Female Sexual Function Index (FSFI): a multidimensional self-report instrument for the assessment of female sexual function. J Sex Marital Ther 2000;26(2):191–208.

96. Corona G, Jannini EA, Maggi M. Inventories for male and female sexual dysfunctions. Int J Impot Res 2006;18(3):236–50.

97. Jeffery DD, Tzeng JP, Keefe FJ, et al. Initial report of the cancer Patient-Reported Outcomes Measurement Information System (PROMIS) sexual function committee: review of sexual function measures and domains used in oncology. Cancer 2009;115(6):1142–53.

98. Baser RE, Li Y, Carter J. Psychometric validation of the Female Sexual Function Index (FSFI) in cancer survivors. Cancer 2012;118(18):4606–18.

99. Rosen RC, Riley A, Wagner G, et al. The international index of erectile function (IIEF): a multidimensional scale for assessment of erectile dysfunction. Urology 1997;49(6):822–30.

100. Mick J, Hughes M, Cohen MZ. Using the BETTER Model to assess sexuality. Clin J Oncol Nurs 2004;8(1):84–6.

101. Annon JS. The PLISSIT Model: a proposed conceptual scheme for the behavioral treatment of sexual problems. J Sex Educ Ther 1976;2(2):1–15.

102. Bakewell RT, Volker DL. Sexual dysfunction related to the treatment of young women with breast cancer. Clin J Oncol Nurs 2005;9(6):697–702.

103. Darwish-Yassine M, Berenji M, Wing D, et al. Evaluating long-term patient-centered outcomes following prostate cancer treatment: findings from the Michigan Prostate Cancer Survivor study. J Cancer Surviv 2014;8(1):121–30.

104. Park ER, Norris RL, Bober SL. Sexual health communication during cancer care: barriers and recommendations. Cancer J 2009;15(1):74–7.

105. Denton AS, Maher EJ. Interventions for the physical aspects of sexual dysfunction in women following pelvic radiotherapy. Cochrane Database Syst Rev 2003;(1):CD003750.

106. Miles T, Johnson N. Vaginal dilator therapy for women receiving pelvic radiotherapy. Cochrane Database Syst Rev 2010;(9):CD007291.

107. Goldfinger C, Pukall CF, Gentilcore-Saulnier E, et al. A prospective study of pelvic floor physical therapy: pain and psychosexual outcomes in provoked vestibulodynia. J Sex Med 2009;6(7):1955–68.

108. Tu FF, Holt J, Gonzales J, et al. Physical therapy evaluation of patients with chronic pelvic pain: a controlled study. Am J Obstet Gynecol 2008;198(3):272.e1-7.

109. Schroder M, Mell LK, Hurteau JA, et al. Clitoral therapy device for treatment of sexual dysfunction in irradiated cervical cancer patients. Int J Radiat Oncol Biol Phys 2005;61(4):1078–86.

110. Yuan J, Zhang R, Yang Z, et al. Comparative effectiveness and safety of oral phosphodiesterase type 5 inhibitors for erectile dysfunction: a systematic review and network meta-analysis. Eur Urol 2013;63(5):902–12.

111. Carvalheira AA, Pereira NM, Maroco J, et al. Dropout in the treatment of erectile dysfunction with PDE5: a study on predictors and a qualitative analysis of reasons for discontinuation. J Sex Med 2012;9(9):2361–9.

112. Gresser U, Gleiter CH. Erectile dysfunction: comparison of efficacy and side effects of the PDE-5 inhibitors sildenafil, vardenafil and tadalafil–review of the literature. Eur J Med Res 2002;7(10):435–46.

113. Raina R, Lakin MM, Thukral M, et al. Long-term efficacy and compliance of intracorporeal (IC) injection for erectile dysfunction following radical prostatectomy: SHIM (IIEF-5) analysis. Int J Impot Res 2003;15(5):318–22.

114. Dennis RL, McDougal WS. Pharmacological treatment of erectile dysfunction after radical prostatectomy. J Urol 1988;139(4):775–6.

115. Baniel J, Israilov S, Segenreich E, et al. Comparative evaluation of treatments for erectile dysfunction in patients with prostate cancer after radical retropubic prostatectomy. BJU Int 2001;88(1):58–62.

116. Siddons HM, Wootten AC, Costello AJ. A randomised, wait-list controlled trial: evaluation of a cognitive-behavioural group intervention on psycho-sexual adjustment for men with localised prostate cancer. Psychooncology 2013;22(10):2186–92.

117. Badr H, Krebs P. A systematic review and meta-analysis of psychosocial interventions for couples coping with cancer. Psychooncology 2013;22(8):1688–704.

118. Beck AM, Robinson JW, Carlson LE. Sexual intimacy in heterosexual couples after prostate cancer treatment: what we know and what we still need to learn. Urol Oncol 2009;27(2):137–43.

119. Chambers SK, Pinnock C, Lepore SJ, et al. A systematic review of psychosocial interventions for men with prostate cancer and their partners. Patient Educ Couns 2011;85(2):e75–88.

120. Chisholm KE, McCabe MP, Wootten AC, et al. Review: psychosocial interventions addressing sexual or relationship functioning in men with prostate cancer. J Sex Med 2012;9(5):1246–60.

121. Chambers SK, Schover L, Halford K, et al. ProsCan for Couples: a feasibility study for evaluating peer support within a controlled research design. Psychooncology 2013;22(2):475–9.

122. Zhou ES, Kim Y, Rasheed M, et al. Marital satisfaction of advanced prostate cancer survivors and their spousal caregivers: the dyadic effects of physical and mental health. Psychooncology 2011;20(12):1353–7.

123. Badr H, Taylor CL. Sexual dysfunction and spousal communication in couples coping with prostate cancer. Psychooncology 2009;18(7):735–46.

124. Garos S, Kluck A, Aronoff D. Prostate cancer patients and their partners: differences in satisfaction indices and psychological variables. J Sex Med 2007;4(5): 1394–403.

125. Soloway CT, Soloway MS, Kim SS, et al. Sexual, psychological and dyadic qualities of the prostate cancer 'couple'. BJU Int 2005;95(6):780–5.

126. Scott JL, Halford WK, Ward BG. United we stand? The effects of a couple-coping intervention on adjustment to early stage breast or gynecological cancer. J Consult Clin Psychol 2004;72(6):1122–35.

127. Manne SL, Ostroff JS, Winkel G, et al. Couple-focused group intervention for women with early stage breast cancer. J Consult Clin Psychol 2005;73(4): 634–46.

128. Zhou ES, Bober SL, Nekhlyudov L, et al. Physical and emotional health information needs and preferences of long-term prostate cancer survivors. Patient Educ Couns 2016;99(12):2049–54.

129. Hordern A, Street A. Issues of intimacy and sexuality in the face of cancer: the patient perspective. Cancer Nurs 2007;30(6):E11–8.

130. Bourgeois-Law G, Lotocki R. Sexuality and gynecological cancer: a needs assessment. Can J Hum Sex 1999;8:231–40.

131. Feldman-Stewart D, Brundage MD, Hayter C, et al. What questions do patients with curable prostate cancer want answered? Med Decis Making 2000;20(1): 7–19.

132. Mercadante S, Vitrano V, Catania V. Sexual issues in early and late stage cancer: a review. Support Care Cancer 2010;18(6):659–65.

133. Stead ML, Brown JM, Fallowfield L, et al. Lack of communication between healthcare professionals and women with ovarian cancer about sexual issues. Br J Cancer 2003;88(5):666–71.

134. Park ER, Bober SL, Campbell EG, et al. General internist communication about sexual function with cancer survivors. J Gen Intern Med 2009;24(Suppl 2): S407–11.

Diet, Physical Activity, and Body Weight in Cancer Survivorship

Karishma Mehra, MD, Alyssa Berkowitz, MPH, Tara Sanft, MD*

KEYWORDS

- Cancer • Survivorship • Obesity • Diet • Exercise

KEY POINTS

- There is increasing evidence of the role of dietary patterns and prognosis in cancer survivors.
- In many cancer types, obesity and cancer incidence, recurrence, and cancer-specific mortality have been linked.
- Physical activity in cancer survivors has been associated with an improvement in quality of life and cancer recurrence.
- There are ongoing research efforts to understand the role of diet, physical activity, and body weight in cancer survivorship.
- Diet and physical activity recommendations for cancer survivors do exist.

INTRODUCTION

The World Health Organization and the American Cancer Society (ACS) recommend cancer survivors consume a plant-based diet and participate in 150 minutes of moderate intensity exercise per week.[1] Lifestyle modification has been shown to have benefits in cancer prevention, risk reduction, and factors that contribute to quality of life (QOL). This review is divided into 3 lifestyle-related categories: diet, obesity, and physical activity. Within each topic, the authors focus on the information for the most commonly studied cancer sites and include information on emerging data for other cancer sites as appropriate.

DIET

Differences in dietary patterns have long been thought to contribute to variation in cancer incidence throughout the world.[2] Although concern about the dietary intake and

---

Disclosure Statement: The authors have nothing to disclose.
Department of Medical Oncology, Yale School of Medicine, 333 Cedar Street, New Haven, CT 06520, USA
* Corresponding author. 300 George Street Suite 120, New Haven, CT.
E-mail address: Tara.sanft@yale.edu

Med Clin N Am 101 (2017) 1151–1165
http://dx.doi.org/10.1016/j.mcna.2017.06.004
0025-7125/17/© 2017 Elsevier Inc. All rights reserved.

medical.theclinics.com

the risk of cancer dates back to the early 1900s,[3] it is in the last 2 decades that epidemiologic studies have shown a definitive link between diet and both incidence and prognosis of cancer. Diet is now considered a modifiable risk in the development of certain cancers.

Breast Cancer

Many observational studies have looked at the relationship between diet and the risk of recurrence and death in breast cancer survivors.[4] Although individual studies have suggested an association between a specific dietary elements like dietary fat, vegetable, fruits, whole grain, and micronutrients and breast cancer risk, results have not been consistent, and most of the available data do not support a strong association between dietary intake and either breast cancer risk or prognosis.[5] A modest increase in breast cancer risk has been associated with regular consumption of alcohol; however, additional interventional studies are required to assess if reduction in alcohol intake will decrease risk or improve outcomes in breast cancer.[6]

Multiple observational studies have looked at dietary fat content and the outcomes of breast cancer.[5] Systematic reviews that included observational studies found a nonsignificant trend toward worse prognosis associated with higher dietary fat.[4,5,7] Similarly, no significant association has been found between breast cancer and intake of carbohydrates, fruit and vegetables, soy products, antioxidants, dairy products, and green tea.[8] The absence of statistically significant association may be due to the inherent difficulty in assessing nutrition because studies depend on subject's recall of dietary intake and their compliance with a specific diet. Food itself is complex with multiple nutrients that may interact with each other synergistically to effect the biology of cancer, therefore making it difficult to assess the role of a single dietary factor in cancer risk and prognosis.[9]

Two large randomized trials looked at the effects of dietary modifications on outcomes in early breast cancer. The Women's Interventional Nutrition Study (WINS) enrolled 2437 women with stages I to IIIa breast cancer within 1 year from surgery and randomized them to a low-fat dietary intervention or usual care control group. At 5.6-years follow-up, a significant improvement in disease-free survival was seen in the intervention group, with a relapse rate of 9.8% in the intervention group and 12.4% in the control group (hazard ratio [HR] 0.76, 95% confidence interval [CI] $= 0.06$–0.98, $P = .034$ for adjusted Cox model analysis).[9] At 108 months, a survival analysis was completed based on death registry information and, although the intervention group had few deaths (HR 0.82, 95% CI 0.64–1.07, $P = .146$), it did not reach statistical significance.[10] However, a subset analysis showed a significant improvement in overall survival in the hormone receptor–negative group.[11] The Women's Healthy Eating and Living (WHEL) study looked at the impact of a low-fat, high fruit and vegetable diet on disease-free survival in 3088 women with stages I to IIIa breast cancer diagnosed in the past 4 years. At 7-year follow-up, no significant difference was seen in disease-free survival between the groups.[12] An important difference between the WINS study and the WHEL study is that the WINS intervention group saw an average 6-pound weight loss and the reduction in dietary fat intake was maintained throughout 60 months mean follow-up. The WHEL study was not associated with either weight loss or sustained decrease in dietary fat throughout 6-year follow-up.

Although the relationship between breast cancer outcome and diet has not been clearly established, a randomized trial has shown that a Mediterranean diet with olive oil decreased the risk of development of breast cancer.[13] While this indicates that there may be an association between breast cancer and diet, more randomized studies are required to identify the role of diet modification in breast cancer survivors.

Colorectal Cancer

There is a significant amount of data about the role of diet in the primary prevention of colorectal cancer (CRC). Two prospective cohort studies showed increasing consumption of a western diet (higher intake of red and processed meats, sweets and desserts, French fries, and refined grains) was associated with a significantly increased risk of colon cancer, whereas a prudent diet (higher intake of fruits, vegetables, legumes, fish, poultry, and whole grains) was nonsignificantly associated with a reduced risk.[14,15]

In patients who have been diagnosed with colon cancer, diet patterns have been shown to be associated with cancer-specific outcomes. A study evaluated 1009 patients receiving adjuvant therapy for stage III colon cancer on the CALGB89803 trial. Dietary patterns (western vs prudent) were identified based on questionnaires. During a median follow-up of 5.3 years, significantly worse disease-free survival and overall survival were associated with patients with a higher intake of western diet when compared with the lower quintile of western dietary pattern. In contrast, the prudent dietary pattern was not significantly associated with cancer recurrence or mortality.[16] In a follow-up study the investigators examined the influence of glycemic load and carbohydrate intake on colon cancer. Higher glycemic load and carbohydrate intake were both associated with significantly increased risk of recurrence and mortality in patients with stage III colon cancer,[17] whereas increased coffee consumption of greater than 4 cups per day was shown to reduce the recurrence and mortality risk when compared with never drinkers.[18] Although these studies do suggest a relation between diet and colon cancer outcome, the studies were observational and performed on the same cohort of patients. Additional interventional studies are required to validate this data.

Prostate Cancer

There is more than a 60-fold difference in age-adjusted incidence rates between population groups with the highest (African American men in the United States) and the lowest (Japanese and Chinese men living in their native countries) incidence of prostate cancer.[19] Although part of this may be explained by differences in screening practices, the geographic differences in the incidence of prostate cancer were apparent even before the introduction of prostate-specific antigen (PSA) screening.[20] These geographical differences highlights the potential role of environmental factors, including diet and physical activity in the risk and prognosis of prostate cancer.

A 2015 review identified 44 randomized controlled trials (RCTs) of lifestyle interventions, with prostate cancer progression or mortality outcomes. The included trials involved 3418 patients with prostate cancer from 13 countries. In the review, a trial of a nutritional supplement of pomegranate seed, green tea, broccoli, and turmeric; a 4-arm randomized trial comparing usual diet with or without flaxseed supplementation versus low-fat diet with or without flaxseed; and a trial supplementing soy, lycopene, selenium, and coenzyme Q10, all demonstrated beneficial effects.[21] Another review from 2011 including all literature studying the effects of macronutrients and micronutrients in the outcome of prostate cancer[22] showed that there was evidence linking worse outcomes in prostate cancer with high fat content and possible benefits of coffee and lycopene. Reviewers concluded that most studies were small and heterogeneous, and therefore no specific recommendations could be made. However, they suggested a "heart healthy equals prostate healthy" approach may be used to counsel patients about diet.

The MEAL (Men's Eating and Living) study was a feasibility study that tested a telephone-based intervention to increase the intake of vegetables in patients with early-stage prostate cancer. Men in the intervention arm increased daily intake of total vegetables, and fat intake was decreased.[23] A phase 3 trial with the same name is currently underway studying the impact of the above intervention on PSA progression.

Other Cancers

Although most data exist for breast, prostate, and colorectal cancers, smaller observational studies have shown the trends of improved outcomes with fruit and vegetable intake in head and neck cancers,[24] ovarian, endometrial, and bladder cancer.[25]

Many ongoing trials like the Lifestyle Intervention of oVarian cancer (LIVES) trial for ovarian cancer and BLENDS (BLadder cancer, Epidemiology, and Nutritional Determinants) study for bladder cancer are ongoing to study association of dietary factors with incidence and outcomes. Based on the existing data, the National Comprehensive Cancer Network Survivorship guidelines outline diet recommendations in cancer survivors (**Box 1**).

OBESITY

Obesity has been a well-established risk factor for many cancers. In a prospective study of more than 900,000 US adults who were followed more than 16 years, the heaviest members (body mass index [BMI] >40) had a death rate from all cancers 52% (men) and 62% (women) higher than matched men and women of normal weight.

Box 1
National Comprehensive Cancer Network guidelines for cancer survivors

Diet

- Recommended food volumes
  - Vegetables and fruits should comprise half the volume of food on the plate (30% vegetables, 20% fruits)
  - Whole grains should comprise 30% of the plate
  - Protein should comprise 20% of the plate
- Sources of dietary components
  - Fat: plant sources, such as olive or canola oil, avocados, seeds and nuts, and fatty fish
  - Carbohydrates: vegetables, fruits, whole grains, and legumes
  - Protein: poultry, fish, legumes, low-fat dairy foods, and nuts
- Limit intake of red or processed meat and refined sugars

Exercise

- Overall volume of weekly activity should be at least 150 min of moderate intensity activity or 75 min of vigorous intensity activity or equivalent combination
- Two or 3 sessions per week of strength training that include major muscle groups
- Stretch major muscle groups at least two days per week

General physical activity

- Engage in general physical activity daily (eg, taking the stairs, parking in the back of parking lot)
- Physical activity includes exercise, daily routine activities, and recreational activities
- Avoid prolonged sedentary behavior (eg, sitting for long periods)

Data from NCCN Clinical Practice Guidelines in Oncology-Survivorship Version 2.2017. Available at: https://www.nccn.org/professionals/physician_gls/pdf/survivorship.pdf. Accessed July 26, 2017.

Higher BMIs were significantly associated with higher rates of death due to cancer of the esophagus, colon, rectum, liver, gallbladder, pancreas, kidney, non-Hodgkin lymphoma, and multiple myeloma. Increasing risk of death with higher BMI values were observed from cancers of the stomach and prostate in men and from cancers of the breast, uterus, cervix, and ovary in women.[26] Observational studies have shown that obesity at time of diagnosis of cancer is also associated with an increased risk of cancer recurrence and cancer-related mortality. Obesity has been linked with increased risk of toxicities from chemotherapy, increased surgical complications, and higher risk of second malignancies.[27]

Breast Cancer

The relationship between body weight and breast cancer risk is highly dependent on menopausal status. Premenopausal women who are overweight or obese have been shown to have a lower risk of breast cancer as compared with leaner women, whereas the opposite is true in postmenopausal women. A pooled analysis of 7 prospective cohort studies, including 337,819 women and 4385 incident cases of breast cancer, demonstrated that premenopausal women with a BMI greater than 31 kg/m^2 had a relative risk (RR) for breast cancer of 0.54 (95% CI 0.34–0.85) compared with those with a BMI less than 21 kg/m^2. In postmenopausal women, those with a BMI greater than 28 kg/m^2 had an RR of 1.26 (95% CI 1.09–1.46) compared with women with a BMI less than 21 kg/m^2.[28] The risk of breast cancer in obese postmenopausal women may be especially pronounced in those who gain a significant amount of weight during adulthood.[29] Several meta-analyses have shown a significant decrease in overall survival and breast cancer–free survival in obese versus nonobese patients regardless of age, stage, menopausal status, or hormone receptor status,[30,31] and obesity is associated with increased risk of recurrence and death by about 35% to 40%.[32]

Two large intervention studies, Lifestyle Intervention Study for Adjuvant Treatment of Early Breast Cancer (LISA) and Exercise and Nutrition to Enhance Recovery and Good Health for You (ENERGY), looking at weight loss and breast cancer have been completed. However, they were not designed to study the effects of weight loss on breast cancer recurrence and cancer specific mortality. The LISA study randomly assigned 338 postmenopausal women with hormone receptor–positive breast cancer to a 2-year telephone-based weight loss intervention or to usual care. Although the primary end point of the LISA trial was effect of weight loss on disease-free survival, the study was terminated due to lack of funding and was not able to accrue the required sample size to answer that question. It did, however, find women randomized to the intervention group lost more weight than controls and also reported significant improvements in physical functioning scores.[33] Similarly, the ENERGY Trial randomized 692 women with a history of breast cancer to a group-based weight loss program or to a less intensive control group that received 2 meetings with a dietitian and nontargeted print materials.[34] The study showed significant decrease in weight and lower blood pressure in the interventional group when compared with the less intensive group. This trial was not powered to study the effect of weight loss on breast cancer outcomes. The LEAN study (Lifestyle, Exercise, And Nutrition) was an RCT of 100 breast cancer survivors who were randomly assigned to 1 of 3 arms: an in-person weight loss program, a telephone-based weight loss program, or usual care. In addition to a 6% average weight loss, patients in both the in-person and the telephone-based intervention groups also had a 30% decrease in C-reactive protein versus 1% in the control group. C-reactive protein, a marker of inflammation, has been implicated in reduced survival in breast cancer.[35] Those women who experienced greater than 5% weight loss were found to have significant decreases in insulin, leptin, and interleukin-6 (IL-6), biomarkers found to be associated with worse breast cancer risk and mortality.[36]

Two large-scale trials in Europe the DIANA-V (Docetaxel and androgens V study)[37] and SUCCESS-C (Simultaneous Study of Docetaxel Gemcitabine combination adjuvant treatment as well as Extended Bisphosphonate and Surveillance Trial–C)[38] looking at the impact of lifestyle intervention upon breast cancer outcomes have completed accrual, and results are anticipated. In the United States and Canada, the BWEL study (Breast Cancer Weight Loss), a phase 3 randomized trial evaluating the impact of a 2-year telephone-based weight loss intervention on invasive disease-free survival in overweight and obese women with stage II or III breast cancer, is underway and started enrollment in 2016.

Colon Cancer

In nonmetastatic colon cancer, the relationship between BMI and time to recurrence is often J-shaped, such that patients who are underweight (BMI <18.5 kg/m^2) or with class II or III obesity (BMI $\geq$35 kg/m^2) have poorer prognosis when compared with those with a BMI between 18.5 and 35 kg/m^2. Furthermore, there is an obesity paradox in colon cancer, such that patients who are overweight (BMI 25.0–29.9) tend to have superior outcomes compared with those of a normal weight.[39] This relationship between BMI and CRC outcome is modified by gender. In both colon and rectal cancer, obese men have an increased risk of recurrence or death when compared with men with normal weight; however, no such relationship was seen in obese women. The difference in risk based on gender is likely explained by differences in storage of excess adiposity between men (abdominal region) and women (lower extremities), given waist circumference is independently associated with cancer recurrence and death.[40] At this time, it is unclear if the relationship between obesity and colon cancer is causal and, to the authors' knowledge, no studies have been undertaken to look at the effect of alteration in weight to colon cancer outcomes.

Prostate Cancer

Many studies have explored the risk and outcome of prostate cancer in relation to obesity. Both elevated BMI and waist circumference/abdominal adiposity have been associated with risk of advanced prostate cancer.[41,42] A pooled analysis of cohorts from Norway, Sweden, and Austria found no higher risk of prostate cancer in men with the metabolic syndrome, but the risk of prostate cancer death was higher due to the underlying associations with BMI and high blood pressure.[43] For men who underwent a radical prostatectomy, a positive association was found between increased BMI and biochemical recurrence.[44]

Recently, 2 prospective cohort studies examining the incidence and mortality of prostate cancer in Danish men showed that obesity was not associated with an increased risk of prostate cancer; however, obese men tended to be diagnosed with more advanced cancer (48% vs 37% incidence of stage III/IV cancer in obese vs nonobese men, $P = .006$). Obese men with prostate cancer had significantly higher prostate cancer–specific mortality even after adjusting for stage, suggesting a stage-independent causal pathway where prostate cancer in obese men has higher fatality, even in early-stage disease.[45]

Other Cancer

Obesity has also been linked to both risk and outcomes of various other malignancies. Risk of development of many solid tumors like esophageal, gastric, melanoma, pancreatic, and hepatocellular carcinoma has been linked to obesity.[46] In hematologic malignancies, obese patients have been shown to have a worse prognosis with lymphoma, multiple myeloma, and leukemia. In multiple myeloma, obesity is also implicated as an etiologic risk.[47] In renal cancers, although obesity is an associated risk factor,[48] the effect of obesity on outcomes may differ by histologic subtype and needs further investigation.[49]

In female cancer survivors, obesity has been shown to correlate with worse prognosis of both endometrial and ovarian cancer.[50] The LIVES (Lifestyle Intervention for Ovarian Cancer Enhanced Survival trial) trial will randomly assign patients with ovarian cancer to receive a 2-year lifestyle intervention (primarily delivered via telephone) or usual care, with the primary outcome of progression-free survival (PFS).[51]

EXERCISE

Because of the complexity of cancer as a disease and the extensive variety of treatment options, there are several ways that physical activity can interact with the large number of "cancer variables." Courneya constructed the following framework of 4 propositions to conceptualize the different interactions between physical activity and cancer variables: (1) Cancer variables may be outcomes of physical activity, (2) Cancer variables may be moderators of physical activity outcomes, (3) Cancer variables may be determinants of physical activity, and (4) Cancer variables may be moderators of physical activity determinants.[52] Both observational and interventional studies have demonstrated the effect of physical activity in cancer survivorship, with most data coming from breast, colorectal, and prostate cancer survivors.

Breast Cancer

Breast cancer is the most researched cancer type in the field of exercise oncology. In 2005 data from the Nurses' Health Study showed that survivors who participated in 3 h/wk of moderate-intense physical activity after diagnosis had a 50% lower risk of recurrence, breast cancer–specific death, and all-cause mortality.[53] These findings were supported by a 2012 systematic review of 6 observational studies that found that physical activity was associated with a significant decrease of breast cancer–related mortality, ranging from 41% to 51%.[54] Included in the systematic review was The Collaborative Women's Longevity Study,[54,55] an observational study of 4482 breast cancer survivors, demonstrating that moderate-intensity activity was associated with a lower risk of breast cancer–specific death and that performing 5 MET-h/wk (metabolic equivalent task-hours per week) of moderate-intensity activity reduced the risk of breast cancer–specific death by 15%.[55] In addition, the HEAL (Health, Eating, Activity, and Lifestyle) study examined 933 breast cancer survivors and found that women 2 years after diagnosis who reported participating in recreational physical activity of at least 9 MET-h/wk had 64% to 67% lower risk of all-cause mortality than those who were inactive (P for trend = .0046).[56]

Several studies have demonstrated the association between exercise among breast cancer survivors and QOL. A meta-analysis of 3 studies found that exercise was associated with an improvement of 4 points on the Functional Assessment of Cancer Therapy (FACT) questionnaire, which is clinically meaningful for QOL.[57] Results from the BEAT Cancer (Better Exercise Adherence after Treatment for Cancer)[58] intervention found that participating in a 3-month exercise intervention was associated with improved physical health composite scores, mental health composite scores, and each subscore category. Significance between group differences in the mental health composite score, vitality subscore, and mental health subscore continued to be seen at the 3-month postintervention time point.[58] Exercise may also help alleviate side effects associated with aromatase inhibitor (AI) use in breast cancer survivors. In an RCT conducted by Irwin and colleagues,[59] 121 breast cancer survivors who were currently taking an AI and experiencing arthralgia were randomized to either a 12-month exercise program or to usual care. Over the 12 months, statistically significant decreases in joint pain scores, pain severity, and pain interference were observed between exercisers versus the usual-care group. In addition, statistically significant improvements in both lower-extremity joint pain symptoms and upper-extremity physical function were seen among women in the intervention group.[59]

Several studies have examined the mechanisms that exercise impacts in breast cancer survivors. A meta-analysis of 5 randomized trials of breast cancer survivors who had been diagnosed with stage I-IIIA cancer found that exercise was associated with a moderate reduction in insulin-like growth factor-I and significantly improved serum concentration levels of both insulin-like growth factors binding protein-I (IGFBP-I) and IGFBP-III.[60]

Colorectal Cancer

A 2012 systematic review of studies conducted in CRC survivors found that among the 5 observational studies where postdiagnosis physical activity was examined, physical activity was associated with a statistically significant reduced risk in all-cause mortality ranging from 23% to 63%.[54,61-65] The systematic review included a study of 832 stage III colon cancer survivors that found that participating in approximately 300 min/wk of postdiagnosis physical activity was associated with a 45% to 49% increase in disease-free survival.[63] Using data from the Health Professionals Follow-up Study, Meyerhardt and colleagues[64] also found that when compared with those who reported ≤ 3 MET-h/wk of physical activity, male survivors who reported ≥ 27 MET-h/wk had an adjusted HR of 0.47 (95% CI, 0.24–0.92) and 0.59 (95% 0.41–0.86) for CRC-specific and overall mortality, respectively.

Numerous studies have demonstrated that exercise is associated with improved QOL factors among CRC survivors. A Dutch prospective-observational study of more than 1200 CRC survivors found that patient who did not meet the Dutch physical activity guidelines had significantly lower scores on all of the EORTC QLQ-C30 subscales, a questionnaire that measure several HRQoL.[66] In addition, an increase of 1 hour of moderate-vigorous physical activity per week was associated with an increase in the global QOL, physical functioning, role functioning, emotional functioning, cognitive function, and social functioning subscale.[66]

CRC survivors often suffer various disease and treatment side effects, such as bowel dysfunction and fatigue, which can impair their ability to perform physical activities.[67] In an observational study of 479 CRC survivors, the presence of a perceived physical activity barrier was associated with a decrease in physical activity.[68] Fatigue was the most common barrier reported for not meeting physical activity guidelines, reported by 13% of patients. Participants also reported general aches and pains (10%), difficulty breathing/chronic lung comorbidities (10%), and lack of time (8%) as barriers to physical activity.[68] These results are consistent with previous findings by Courneya and colleagues,[69] who found that lack of time, nonspecific treatment side effects, and fatigue were the most common reasons participants gave for not adhering to their intervention exercise regime. The CHALLENGE (Colon Health Life-long Exercise Change) study aimed to address ways to increase CRC survivors' physical activity by randomizing 273 survivors into a structured exercise program (SEP) cohort or a health education materials (HEM) cohort. Although both groups increased their physical activity from baseline to 1 year, those in the SEP group had on average a 10.5 MET-h/wk greater increase than the HEM cohort (95% CI, 3.1–17.9 $P = .002$).[70]

The COURAGE trial (Colon Recurrence and Aerobic Exercise) is an ongoing randomized study examining the impact of exercise among 39 nonmetastatic CRC survivors. The primary objective of the study is to measure the feasibility (adherence rates), safety (adverse events), and physiologic impact (prognostic biomarkers) of low-dose aerobic exercise, high-dose aerobic exercise, or usual-care among this population.[71]

Two RCTs found that moderate-intensity physical activity decreased urinary 8-oxo-2'-deoxyguanosine excretion, a biomarker of oxidative DNA damage, and reduced circulating levels of lipopolysaccharide-stimulated IL-1.[54,72,73]

Prostate Cancer

Several different studies have examined the impact of postdiagnosis physical activity on survival rates among prostate cancer survivors. Kenfield and colleagues[74] examined the physical activity of 2705 prostate cancer survivors and found that men who engaged in $\geq$3 h/wk of vigorous activity had a 49% reduction in all-cause mortality and a 61% reduction in prostate cancer–specific mortality when compared with men who performed less than 1 h/wk of vigorous activity. Another study that examined 1455 prostate cancer survivors found that men who walked at a brisk pace $\geq$3 h/wk had a 57% statistically significant lower risk of cancer progression compared with men who did not, even when controlled for BMI.[75] A third study examined 4623 prostate cancer survivors who had localized disease for up to 15 years. Engaging in $\geq$20 min/d versus less than 20 min/d of postdiagnosis moderate walking/bicycling was associated with a 39% reduced risk of disease-specific mortality and engaging in $\geq$1 versus less than 1 h/wk of moderate-vigorous exercise was associated with a 32% lower risk of disease-specific mortality.[76] In all of these studies, men who were in the highest categories of physical activities tended to be younger, less likely to smoke, and have a lower BMI.

Physical activity has also been shown to improve QOL and physical functioning among prostate cancer survivors.[77] Galvao and colleagues[78] found that survivors who were inactive had higher International Prostate Symptoms Scores than individuals who were insufficiently active (engaging in physical activity but not meeting recommendations) and sufficiently active (meeting the recommended guidelines). A randomized study of 100 prostate cancer survivors on long-term androgen-deprivation therapy found that those in the exercise intervention arm saw greater clinical relevant improvements in Functional Assessment of Cancer Therapy–Prostate (FACT-P) (P = .0001) and Functional Assessment of Cancer Therapy–Fatigue (FACT-F) (P<.001) scores at 12 weeks (P = .0001).[79]

Other Cancers

There is insufficient literature regarding the impact of physical activity on survival for gynecologic cancer survivors. However, several studies have demonstrated that there is a positive correlation between participating in physical activity and improvement in QOL for this population. There have been a handful of studies that have explored the feasibility of exercise interventions among uterine cancer survivors. The SUCEED (Survivors of Uterine Cancer Empowered by Exercise and Healthy Diet) study randomized 75 overweight endometrial cancer survivors to a lifestyle intervention (consisting of 6-month education and counseling program) or usual care. There was an 84% adherence rate in the intervention group, and women who received the intervention reported performing a significantly greater number of physical activity minutes than the usual care arm.[80] Babatunde and colleagues'[81] systematic review of endometrial cancer survivors found that out of the 7 studies examined, all but one found significant positive association between meeting physical activity guidelines and improved QOL.

A retrospective cohort analysis of 63 endometrial cancer survivors found that individuals who participated in a single-arm exercise intervention reported significant improvements in sexual function scores ($P = .002$).[82] An observational study of 359 ovarian cancer survivors showed that individuals who met or exceeded the ACS recommended guidelines had significantly higher QOL score on the Functional Assessment of Cancer Therapy–Ovarian (FACT-O) than those who did not. In addition, they found that disease status moderates the association between physical activity and QOL, with disease-free participants scoring higher on the FACT-O.[83]

Although there is limited published research on survival and exercise for gynecologic cancers, current studies are being conducted to examine the relationship. As mentioned in the obesity section, The LIVES is a 24-month randomized lifestyle invention examining the impact of a dietary and physical activity on PFS and QOL among stage II-IV ovarian cancer survivors who have completed treatment.[51] In addition, the Diet and Exercise in Uterine Cancer Survivors (DEUS pilot) is phase 2 randomized study testing the feasibility of an 8-week group session healthy eating and physical activity program in endometrial cancer survivors.[84]

There are currently few studies that have examined exercise among lung cancer. Lung cancer has unique comorbidities that effect physical activity participation, such as a decrease in VO_2-max due to lung capacity. A few small studies have found that participating in a rehabilitation program for lung cancer survivors who had undergone surgery that included cycling was associated with improvement in cardiorespiratory fitness.[85] There are studies that are currently ongoing for lung cancer survivors including the POSITIVE study, an RCT for inoperable lung cancer survivors that will examine the effect of a 24-week exercise program on QOL and fatigue.[86]

SUMMARY

As additional data on the benefits of lifestyle modification after cancer continue to emerge, future directions should focus on understanding the biological mechanisms that explain how healthy behaviors lead to improved outcomes; work to investigate this is underway. Perhaps more importantly, future directions should focus on the dissemination and implementation of successful strategies to help patients make healthy changes that can be sustained over time.

REFERENCES

1. Rock CL, Doyle C, Demark-Wahnefried W, et al. Nutrition and physical activity guidelines for cancer survivors. CA Cancer J Clin 2012;62:243–74.
2. Alcantara EN, Speckmann EW. Diet, nutrition, and cancer. Am J Clin Nutr 1976; 29:1035–47.
3. Cancer and diet. Am J Public Health (N Y) 1924;14:53–5.
4. Goodwin PJ, Ennis M, Pritchard KI, et al. Diet and breast cancer: evidence that extremes in diet are associated with poor survival. J Clin Oncol 2003;21:2500–7.
5. Rock CL, Demark-Wahnefried W. Nutrition and survival after the diagnosis of breast cancer: a review of the evidence. J Clin Oncol 2002;20:3302–16.
6. Key TJ, Reeves GK. Alcohol, diet, and risk of breast cancer. BMJ 2016;353:i2503.
7. Patterson RE, Cadmus LA, Emond JA, et al. Physical activity, diet, adiposity and female breast cancer prognosis: a review of the epidemiologic literature. Maturitas 2010;66:5–15.
8. Michels KB, Mohllajee AP, Roset-Bahmanyar E, et al. Diet and breast cancer: a review of the prospective observational studies. Cancer 2007;109:2712–49.

9. Mayne ST, Playdon MC, Rock CL. Diet, nutrition, and cancer: past, present and future. Nat Rev Clin Oncol 2016;13:504–15.

10. Chlebowski RT, Blackburn GL, Hoy MK, et al. Survival analyses from the Women's Intervention Nutrition Study (WINS) evaluating dietary fat reduction and breast cancer outcome. J Clin Oncol 2008;26:522.

11. Chlebowski RT, Blackburn GL, Thomson CA, et al. Dietary fat reduction and breast cancer outcome: interim efficacy results from the Women's Intervention Nutrition Study. J Natl Cancer Inst 2006;98:1767–76.

12. Pierce JP, Natarajan L, Caan BJ, et al. Influence of a diet very high in vegetables, fruit, and fiber and low in fat on prognosis following treatment for breast cancer: the women's healthy eating and living (WHEL) randomized trial. JAMA 2007;298: 289–98.

13. Toledo E, Salas-Salvado J, Donat-Vargas C, et al. Mediterranean diet and invasive breast cancer risk among women at high cardiovascular risk in the PRE-DIMED trial: a randomized clinical trial. JAMA Intern Med 2015;175:1752–60.

14. Fung T, Hu FB, Fuchs C, et al. Major dietary patterns and the risk of colorectal cancer in women. Arch Intern Med 2003;163:309–14.

15. Wu K, Hu FB, Fuchs C, et al. Dietary patterns and risk of colon cancer and adenoma in a cohort of men (United States). Cancer Causes Control 2004;15: 853–62.

16. Meyerhardt JA, Stuart K, Fuchs CS, et al. Phase II study of FOLFOX, bevacizumab and erlotinib as first-line therapy for patients with metastatic colorectal cancer. Ann Oncol 2007;18:1185–9.

17. Meyerhardt JA, Sato K, Niedzwiecki D, et al. Dietary glycemic load and cancer recurrence and survival in patients with stage III colon cancer: findings from CALGB 89803. J Natl Cancer Inst 2012;104:1702–11.

18. Guercio BJ, Sato K, Niedzwiecki D, et al. Coffee intake, recurrence, and mortality in stage III colon cancer: results from CALGB 89803 (Alliance). J Clin Oncol 2015; 33:3598–607.

19. Wilson KM, Giovannucci EL, Mucci LA. Lifestyle and dietary factors in the prevention of lethal prostate cancer. Asian J Androl 2012;14:365–74.

20. Yu H, Harris RE, Gao YT, et al. Comparative epidemiology of cancers of the colon, rectum, prostate and breast in Shanghai, China versus the United States. Int J Epidemiol 1991;20:76–81.

21. Hackshaw-McGeagh LE, Perry RE, Leach VA, et al. A systematic review of dietary, nutritional, and physical activity interventions for the prevention of prostate cancer progression and mortality. Cancer Causes Control 2015;26:1521–50.

22. Masko EM, Freedland SJ. Prostate cancer and diet: food for thought? BJU Int 2011;107:1359–60.

23. Parsons JK, Newman V, Mohler JL, et al. The men's eating and living (MEAL) study: a cancer and leukemia group B pilot trial of dietary intervention for the treatment of prostate cancer. Urology 2008;72:633–7.

24. Butler C, Lee YA, Li S, et al. Diet and the risk of head-and-neck cancer among never-smokers and smokers in a Chinese population. Cancer Epidemiol 2017; 46:20–6.

25. Stepien M, Chajes V, Romieu I. The role of diet in cancer: the epidemiologic link. Salud Publica Mex 2016;58:261–73.

26. Calle EE, Rodriguez C, Walker-Thurmond K, et al. Overweight, obesity, and mortality from cancer in a prospectively studied cohort of U.S. adults. N Engl J Med 2003;348:1625–38.

27. Ligibel JA. Jennifer Ligibel discusses new data strengthening the link between obesity and cancer. Oncology (Williston Park) 2016;30(11):952, 1007.

28. van den Brandt PA, Spiegelman D, Yaun SS, et al. Pooled analysis of prospective cohort studies on height, weight, and breast cancer risk. Am J Epidemiol 2000; 152:514–27.

29. Ahn J, Schatzkin A, Lacey JV Jr, et al. Adiposity, adult weight change, and post-menopausal breast cancer risk. Arch Intern Med 2007;167:2091–102.

30. Protani M, Coory M, Martin JH. Effect of obesity on survival of women with breast cancer: systematic review and meta-analysis. Breast Cancer Res Treat 2010;123: 627–35.

31. Niraula S, Ocana A, Ennis M, et al. Body size and breast cancer prognosis in relation to hormone receptor and menopausal status: a meta-analysis. Breast Cancer Res Treat 2012;134:769–81.

32. Jiralerspong S, Goodwin PJ. Obesity and breast cancer prognosis: evidence, challenges, and opportunities. J Clin Oncol 2016;34:4203–16.

33. Goodwin PJ, Segal RJ, Vallis M, et al. Randomized trial of a telephone-based weight loss intervention in postmenopausal women with breast cancer receiving letrozole: the LISA trial. J Clin Oncol 2014;32:2231–9.

34. Rock CL, Flatt SW, Byers TE, et al. Results of the exercise and nutrition to enhance recovery and good health for you (ENERGY) trial: a behavioral weight loss intervention in overweight or obese breast cancer survivors. J Clin Oncol 2015;33:3169–76.

35. Harrigan M, Cartmel B, Loftfield E, et al. Randomized trial comparing telephone versus in-person weight loss counseling on body composition and circulating biomarkers in women treated for breast cancer: the lifestyle, exercise, and nutrition (LEAN) study. J Clin Oncol 2016;34:669–76.

36. Hursting SD. Obesity, energy balance, and cancer: a mechanistic perspective. Cancer Treat Res 2014;159:21–33.

37. Villarini A, Pasanisi P, Traina A, et al. Lifestyle and breast cancer recurrences: the DIANA-5 trial. Tumori 2012;98:1–18.

38. Rack B, Andergassen U, Neugebauer J, et al. The German SUCCESS C Study - the first European lifestyle study on breast cancer. Breast Care (Basel) 2010;5: 395–400.

39. Brown JC, Meyerhardt JA. Obesity and energy balance in GI cancer. J Clin Oncol 2016;34:4217–24.

40. Power ML, Schulkin J. Sex differences in fat storage, fat metabolism, and the health risks from obesity: possible evolutionary origins. Br J Nutr 2008;99:931–40.

41. Fowke JH, Motley SS, Concepcion RS, et al. Obesity, body composition, and prostate cancer. BMC Cancer 2012;12:23.

42. Pischon T, Boeing H, Weikert S, et al. Body size and risk of prostate cancer in the European prospective investigation into cancer and nutrition. Cancer Epidemiol Biomarkers Prev 2008;17:3252–61.

43. Haggstrom C, Stocks T, Ulmert D, et al. Prospective study on metabolic factors and risk of prostate cancer. Cancer 2012;118:6199–206.

44. Cao Y, Ma J. Body mass index, prostate cancer-specific mortality, and biochemical recurrence: a systematic review and meta-analysis. Cancer Prev Res (Phila) 2011;4:486–501.

45. Moller H, Roswall N, Van Hemelrijck M, et al. Prostate cancer incidence, clinical stage and survival in relation to obesity: a prospective cohort study in Denmark. Int J Cancer 2015;136:1940–7.

46. Goodwin PJ, Chlebowski RT. Obesity and cancer: insights for clinicians. J Clin Oncol 2016;34:4197–202.

47. Yang L, Drake BF, Colditz GA. Obesity and other cancers. J Clin Oncol 2016;34: 4231–7.

48. Lauby-Secretan B, Scoccianti C, Loomis D, et al. Body fatness and cancer–viewpoint of the IARC working group. N Engl J Med 2016;375:794–8.

49. Lee WK, Hong SK, Lee S, et al. Prognostic value of body mass index according to histologic subtype in nonmetastatic renal cell carcinoma: a large cohort analysis. Clin Genitourin Cancer 2015;13:461–8.

50. Chlebowski RT, Reeves MM. Weight loss randomized intervention trials in female cancer survivors. J Clin Oncol 2016;34:4238–48.

51. Thomson CA, Crane TE, Miller A, et al. A randomized trial of diet and physical activity in women treated for stage II-IV ovarian cancer: rationale and design of the lifestyle intervention for ovarian cancer enhanced survival (LIVES): an NRG oncology/gynecologic oncology group (GOG-225) study. Contemp Clin Trials 2016;49:181–9.

52. Courneya KS. Physical activity and cancer survivorship: a simple framework for a complex field. Exerc Sport Sci Rev 2014;42:102–9.

53. Holmes MD, Chen WY, Feskanich D, et al. Physical activity and survival after breast cancer diagnosis. JAMA 2005;293:2479–86.

54. Ballard-Barbash R, Friedenreich CM, Courneya KS, et al. Physical activity, biomarkers, and disease outcomes in cancer survivors: a systematic review. J Natl Cancer Inst 2012;104:815–40.

55. Holick CN, Newcomb PA, Trentham-Dietz A, et al. Physical activity and survival after diagnosis of invasive breast cancer. Cancer Epidemiol Biomarkers Prev 2008;17:379–86.

56. Irwin ML, Smith AW, McTiernan A, et al. Influence of pre- and postdiagnosis physical activity on mortality in breast cancer survivors: the health, eating, activity, and lifestyle study. J Clin Oncol 2008;26:3958–64.

57. McNeely ML, Campbell KL, Rowe BH, et al. Effects of exercise on breast cancer patients and survivors: a systematic review and meta-analysis. CMAJ 2006;175: 34–41.

58. Rogers LQ, Courneya KS, Anton PM, et al. Effects of the BEAT Cancer physical activity behavior change intervention on physical activity, aerobic fitness, and quality of life in breast cancer survivors: a multicenter randomized controlled trial. Breast Cancer Res Treat 2015;149:109–19.

59. Irwin ML, Cartmel B, Gross CP, et al. Randomized exercise trial of aromatase inhibitor-induced arthralgia in breast cancer survivors. J Clin Oncol 2015;33: 1104–11.

60. Meneses-Echavez JF, Jimenez EG, Rio-Valle JS, et al. The insulin-like growth factor system is modulated by exercise in breast cancer survivors: a systematic review and meta-analysis. BMC Cancer 2016;16:682.

61. Morikawa T, Kuchiba A, Yamauchi M, et al. Association of CTNNB1 (beta-catenin) alterations, body mass index, and physical activity with survival in patients with colorectal cancer. JAMA 2011;305:1685–94.

62. Meyerhardt JA, Ogino S, Kirkner GJ, et al. Interaction of molecular markers and physical activity on mortality in patients with colon cancer. Clin Cancer Res 2009; 15:5931–6.

63. Meyerhardt JA, Heseltine D, Niedzwiecki D, et al. Impact of physical activity on cancer recurrence and survival in patients with stage III colon cancer: findings from CALGB 89803. J Clin Oncol 2006;24:3535–41.

64. Meyerhardt JA, Giovannucci EL, Ogino S, et al. Physical activity and male colorectal cancer survival. Arch Intern Med 2009;169:2102–8.

65. Meyerhardt JA, Giovannucci EL, Holmes MD, et al. Physical activity and survival after colorectal cancer diagnosis. J Clin Oncol 2006;24:3527–34.

66. Husson O, Mols F, Ezendam NPM, et al. Health-related quality of life is associated with physical activity levels among colorectal cancer survivors: a longitudinal, 3-year study of the PROFILES registry. J Cancer Surviv 2015;9:472–80.

67. Fisher A, Wardle J, Beeken RJ, et al. Perceived barriers and benefits to physical activity in colorectal cancer patients. Support Care Cancer 2016;24:903–10.

68. Fisher A, Smith L, Wardle J. Physical activity advice could become part of routine care for colorectal cancer survivors. Future Oncol 2016;12:139–41.

69. Courneya KS, Friedenreich CM, Quinney HA, et al. A longitudinal study of exercise barriers in colorectal cancer survivors participating in a randomized controlled trial. Ann Behav Med 2005;29:147–53.

70. Courneya KS, Vardy JL, O'Callaghan CJ, et al. Effects of a structured exercise program on physical activity and fitness in colon cancer survivors: one year feasibility results from the CHALLENGE trial. Cancer Epidemiol Biomarkers Prev 2016; 25:969–77.

71. Brown JC, Troxel AB, Ky B, et al. A randomized phase II dose-response exercise trial among colon cancer survivors: purpose, study design, methods, and recruitment results. Contemp Clin Trials 2016;47:366–75.

72. Allgayer H, Nicolaus S, Schreiber S. Decreased interleukin-1 receptor antagonist response following moderate exercise in patients with colorectal carcinoma after primary treatment. Cancer Detect Prev 2004;28:208–13.

73. Allgayer H, Owen RW, Nair J, et al. Short-term moderate exercise programs reduce oxidative DNA damage as determined by high-performance liquid chromatography-electrospray ionization-mass spectrometry in patients with colorectal carcinoma following primary treatment. Scand J Gastroenterol 2008;43: 971–8.

74. Kenfield SA, Stampfer MJ, Giovannucci E, et al. Physical activity and survival after prostate cancer diagnosis in the health professionals follow-up study. J Clin Oncol 2011;29:726–32.

75. Richman EL, Kenfield SA, Stampfer MJ, et al. Physical activity after diagnosis and risk of prostate cancer progression: data from the cancer of the prostate strategic urologic research endeavor. Cancer Res 2011;71:3889–95.

76. Bonn SE, Sjolander A, Tillander A, et al. Body mass index in relation to serum prostate-specific antigen levels and prostate cancer risk. Int J Cancer 2016; 139:50–7.

77. Thorsen L, Courneya KS, Stevinson C, et al. A systematic review of physical activity in prostate cancer survivors: outcomes, prevalence, and determinants. Support Care Cancer 2008;16:987–97.

78. Galvao DA, Newton RU, Gardiner RA, et al. Compliance to exercise-oncology guidelines in prostate cancer survivors and associations with psychological distress, unmet supportive care needs, and quality of life. Psychooncology 2015. [Epub ahead of print].

79. Bourke L, Gilbert S, Hooper R, et al. Lifestyle changes for improving disease-specific quality of life in sedentary men on long-term androgen-deprivation therapy for advanced prostate cancer: a randomised controlled trial. Eur Urol 2014; 65:865–72.

80. von Gruenigen V, Frasure H, Kavanagh MB, et al. Survivors of uterine cancer empowered by exercise and healthy diet (SUCCEED): a randomized controlled trial. Gynecol Oncol 2012;125:699–704.

81. Babatunde OA, Adams SA, Orekoya O, et al. Effect of physical activity on quality of life as perceived by endometrial cancer survivors: a systematic review. Int J Gynecol Cancer 2016;26:1727–40.

82. Armbruster SD, Song J, Bradford A, et al. Sexual health of endometrial cancer survivors before and after a physical activity intervention: a retrospective cohort analysis. Gynecol Oncol 2016;143:589–95.

83. Stevinson C, Faught W, Steed H, et al. Associations between physical activity and quality of life in ovarian cancer survivors. Gynecol Oncol 2007;106:244–50.

84. Koutoukidis DA, Beeken RJ, Lopes S, et al. Attitudes, challenges and needs about diet and physical activity in endometrial cancer survivors: a qualitative study. Eur J Cancer Care (Engl) 2016. [Epub ahead of print].

85. Jones LW. Physical activity and lung cancer survivorship. Recent Results Cancer Res 2011;186:255–74.

86. Wiskemann J, Hummler S, Diepold C, et al. POSITIVE study: physical exercise program in non-operable lung cancer patients undergoing palliative treatment. BMC Cancer 2016;16:499.

Screening for Recurrence and Secondary Cancers

Jillian L. Simard, MD[a], Sheetal M. Kircher, MD[b], Aarati Didwania, MD[c],
Mita Sanghavi Goel, MD, MPH[d],*

KEYWORDS

- Cancer survivor • Recurrence surveillance • Secondary cancer screening

KEY POINTS

- As cancer therapies improve, the adult cancer survivor population increases over time; however, these survivors are at increased risk of developing recurrence and secondary cancers.
- Primary care providers are increasingly responsible for monitoring cancer survivors for long-term effects of therapy as well as for cancer recurrence and secondary cancers.
- Tailored plans for surveillance for locoregional recurrence, metastatic recurrence, and secondary cancer development depend on the type of primary malignancy, treatment regimen, and presence of hereditary cancer syndromes.

INTRODUCTION

With an estimated 15 million cancer survivors in 2016 and increasing numbers projected over the next decade, the importance of cancer surveillance and screening for secondary cancers is increasingly relevant (**Fig. 1**). Most individuals with a prior history of cancer are at least 5 years to 10 years postdiagnosis.[1] After treatment of their primary cancers, survivors continue to be at risk for locoregional and metastatic recurrences as well as secondary cancers. Approximately 1 in 12 cancer survivors develops a second primary malignancy at some point.[2] Even though the role of survivor care is falling increasingly on primary care providers (PCPs), many PCPs report feeling ill equipped to adequately manage this population.[3]

Recognizing these challenges, in 2005 the Institute of Medicine published its report "From Cancer Patient to Cancer Survivor: Lost in Transition"[4] to improve awareness of

Disclosures: The authors have nothing to disclose.
[a] Internal Medicine, Northwestern Memorial Hospital, 201 East Huron, Galter 3-150, Chicago, IL 60611, USA; [b] Department of Medicine, Northwestern University Feinberg School of Medicine, 676 North St. Clair, Suite 850, Chicago, IL 60611, USA; [c] Division of General Internal Medicine and Geriatrics, Department of Medicine, Northwestern University Feinberg School of Medicine, 675 North St. Clair Street, 18-200, Chicago, IL 60611, USA; [d] Division of General Internal Medicine and Geriatrics, Department of Medicine, Northwestern University Feinberg School of Medicine, 750 North Lake Shore Drive, 10th Floor, Chicago, IL 60611, USA
* Corresponding author.
E-mail address: mgoel@nm.org

Med Clin N Am 101 (2017) 1167–1180
http://dx.doi.org/10.1016/j.mcna.2017.06.010
0025-7125/17/© 2017 Elsevier Inc. All rights reserved.

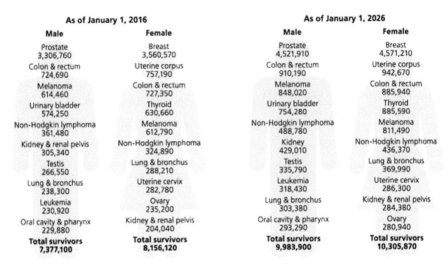

As of January 1, 2016		As of January 1, 2026	
Male	**Female**	**Male**	**Female**
Prostate 3,306,760	Breast 3,560,570	Prostate 4,521,910	Breast 4,571,210
Colon & rectum 724,690	Uterine corpus 757,190	Colon & rectum 910,190	Uterine corpus 942,670
Melanoma 614,460	Colon & rectum 727,350	Melanoma 848,020	Colon & rectum 885,940
Urinary bladder 574,250	Thyroid 630,660	Urinary bladder 754,280	Thyroid 885,590
Non-Hodgkin lymphoma 361,480	Melanoma 612,790	Non-Hodgkin lymphoma 488,780	Melanoma 811,490
Kidney & renal pelvis 305,340	Non-Hodgkin lymphoma 324,890	Kidney 429,010	Non-Hodgkin lymphoma 436,370
Testis 266,550	Lung & bronchus 288,210	Testis 335,790	Lung & bronchus 369,990
Lung & bronchus 238,300	Uterine cervix 282,780	Leukemia 318,430	Uterine cervix 286,300
Leukemia 230,920	Ovary 235,200	Lung & bronchus 303,380	Kidney & renal pelvis 284,380
Oral cavity & pharynx 229,880	Kidney & renal pelvis 204,040	Oral cavity & pharynx 293,290	Ovary 280,940
Total survivors 7,377,100	**Total survivors 8,156,120**	**Total survivors 9,983,900**	**Total survivors 10,305,870**

Fig. 1. Cancer treatment and survivorship statistics, 2016. (*From* Miller KD, Siegel RL, Lin CC, et al. Cancer treatment and survivorship statistics, 2016. CA Cancer J Clin 2016;66[4]:273; with permission.)

survivorship as a distinct phase of cancer care. The National Comprehensive Cancer Network (NCCN) and the American Society of Clinical Oncology (ASCO) subsequently published recommendations for best practices in survivor care.[5,6] A key theme across these reports is the importance of a shared care model between oncologist and PCP, where there is frequent communication between providers both during cancer therapy and after. In this model, the oncologist provides the PCP with a survivorship care plan that includes a summary of the cancer and therapy, a list of potential late effects, and up-to-date recommendations for surveillance for recurrence and late effects.[7] Although survivorship care plans should be informed by expert guidelines, it is equally important to bear in mind patient preferences and functional status. For example, screening tests should only be performed if a patient can tolerate downstream assessment and management. Finally, the screening guidelines discussed in this article pertain to asymptomatic patients; any symptoms concerning for recurrence or secondary malignancy should supersede the guidelines and prompt immediate follow-up testing.

SURVEILLANCE FOR RECURRENCE
Breast Cancer

Breast cancer survivors comprise the largest group of cancer survivors; in the United States alone, there are more than 3.5 million women with a history of invasive breast cancer.[1] The risk of both local and distant recurrence is highest within the first few years of diagnosis but remains appreciable for many years after diagnosis, especially in cases of estrogen receptor–positive tumors.[8] For asymptomatic, average-risk women, ASCO recommends a history and physical examination (H&P) every 3 months to 6 months for the first 3 years after treatment, every 6 months to 12 months for years 4 and 5, and annually thereafter as well as yearly mammography of remaining breasts.[9] The NCCN also recommends yearly mammography.[10] More frequent imaging does not incur an overall survival, disease-free survival, or quality-of-life benefit.[11] Patients also should be educated on signs and symptoms concerning for locoregional recurrence, including new lumps, skin changes, chest pain, changes in breast shape or size, and breast or arm swelling, because these may prompt earlier evaluation.[9] For women who have undergone mastectomy or breast reconstruction, a thorough physical examination is particularly important, because imaging surveillance in these cases is technically challenging.

A subset of patients is at an especially high risk of recurrence or second primary breast tumor, and ASCO advises that they undergo annual breast MRI in addition to the other recommendations.[9] These include patients with known breast cancer susceptibility gene (BRCA) mutations and first-degree relatives of BRCA carriers.[12] Because patients may not have had genetic testing at the time of diagnosis, clinicians should routinely assess for factors that prompt a genetic evaluation. In addition, because genetic testing in constantly evolving, some patients may want to revisit a genetic counselor periodically. Extrapolating from guidelines intended for women without a personal history of breast cancer, the following characteristics should prompt consideration of genetic testing: a personal history of triple-negative breast cancer diagnosed before age 60 and a strong family history of breast, colon, endometrial, ovarian, or peritoneal cancer as delineated by the US Preventive Services Task Force (USPSTF) guidelines.[13]

Family history characteristics that indicate increased risk of developing breast cancer and/or carrying a BRCA mutation:

- Breast cancer diagnosed before age 50
- Cancer in both breasts in the same woman
- Both breast and ovarian cancers in either the same woman or the same family
- Multiple breast cancers
- Two or more primary types of BRCA–1-related or BRCA–2-related cancers in a single family member
- Any cases of male breast cancer
- Ashkenazi Jewish ethnicity

Prostate Cancer

As of 2015, there were 3.3 million prostate cancer survivors in the United States, accounting for approximately half of all total male cancer survivors. Most men (92%) are diagnosed at a localized stage.[1] For men with localized disease who pursued definitive therapy with radical prostatectomy and/or radiation therapy, the hallmark of surveillance is the prostate-specific antigen (PSA) level. The NCCN, American Cancer Society (ACS), and ASCO all recommend PSA testing every 6 months to 12 months for the first 5 years after diagnosis and annually thereafter. Unless the PSA level is undetectable, an annual digital rectal examination (DRE) is also recommended.[14–16] Imaging studies are not indicated unless the patient has specific symptoms concerning for recurrence.

The following PSA trends could herald recurrence and should prompt referral back to the primary treating specialist for further evaluation: (1) serum PSA greater than or equal to 2 ng/mL in patients who have undergone radical prostatectomy,[17] (2) a rise of serum PSA greater than or equal to 2 ng/mL above the nadir PSA in patients who have received radiation therapy, and (3) a confirmed PSA rise not yet greater than or equal to 2 ng/mL above the nadir but in young, otherwise healthy men who would be candidates for salvage therapy.[18] Practitioners should reassure patients that a rising PSA does not always indicate recurrent disease necessitating treatment. Some patients treated with radiation experience a self-limited PSA bounce in the first few years after treatment.[19] In these cases, the PSA can be repeated in 3 months to confirm rising levels prior to referral back to the primary treating specialist. Furthermore, many patients experience a biochemical recurrence (rise in PSA) years before any clinical manifestations emerge. Hence, the decision to pursue any salvage therapies takes into account myriad factors, including overall life expectancy.[20]

For men with nodal or metastatic prostate cancer, the NCCN recommends a physical examination and PSA level every 3 months to 6 months as well as a bone scan every 6 months to 12 months.[14] Symptoms concerning for new bony involvement, such as new neurologic deficits or pathologic fractures, should prompt earlier evaluation. Finally, selected patients with localized, low-risk disease can pursue an initial strategy of active surveillance instead of definitive treatment.

Colorectal Cancer

The prevalence of colorectal cancer survivors was an estimated 1.4 million at the end of 2015.[1] Recurrence rates for locally advanced colorectal cancer can be upwards of 40% despite treatment with surgery, chemotherapy, and/or radiation.[21] Surveillance aims to detect both recurrent and new primary tumors, with the premise that early detection makes subsequent curative intervention more likely and improves overall survival.[22] The NCCN, ACS, and ACSO all recommend intensive surveillance during the first 5 years after treatment. Ultimately, the surveillance strategy should be guided by these recommendations but also be informed by patient preference and functional status as well as overall risk of recurrence. Factors that can place a patient at higher risk of recurrence include lymph node involvement, vascular or perineural invasion, poorly differentiated histology, bowel obstruction or localized perforation, and close or positive resection margins.[23–26]

All patients, regardless of stage, should undergo colonoscopy 1 year after resection (or within 3–6 months if the initial colonoscopy was not performed or limited by lumen obstruction). If an advanced (villous polyp, polyp greater than 1 cm, or high-grade dysplasia) adenoma is seen, colonoscopy should be repeated in 1 year; otherwise, colonoscopy can be repeated at 3 years and then every 5 years. Patients with stages II to IV disease should have an H&P, carcinoembryonic antigen (CEA) level, and proctoscopy plus endoscopic ultrasound or MRI (only for rectal cancer not treated with radiation) every 3 months to 6 months for 2 years, then every 6 months for the next 3 years. Finally, CT of the chest, abdomen, and pelvis with intravenous and oral contrast is recommended every 6 months to 12 months for 3 years to 5 years for stages II to III and every 3 months to 6 months for stage IV disease. The role for routine CEA testing or imaging after 5 years is unclear.

Melanoma

An estimated 1.2 million people in the United States have a history of melanoma. There is scant evidence indicating the optimal follow-up of melanoma survivors and no true consensus among the many expert panels.[27–29] It is generally agreed on that all survivors should undergo lifelong annual skin and lymph node examinations to detect early local recurrence and second primary tumors. Up to 8% of survivors develop a second primary melanoma, and this can occur several years after the first melanoma is discovered. In the first 5 years after diagnosis, more frequent clinical visits are recommended, and the frequency can be guided by the estimated risk of recurrence. This risk can be influenced by disease stage, a patient's family history, the presence of other suspicious nevi, and a patient's anticipated ability to detect early signs of recurrence. A large percentage of local recurrences are first detected by patients or their family members, so education on monthly self-examination of the skin and regional lymph nodes is also important.[30]

Historically, there has been less emphasis on surveillance imaging because it was unclear whether early detection of metastatic disease translates into improved survival. This may change since the advent of more effective therapies for metastatic disease, such as immunotherapy. Currently, the NCCN advises providers to consider chest radiograph and CT with or without PET every 3 months to 12 months and annual brain MRI for stages IIB to IV disease. Providers can also consider surveillance ultrasound of the lymph nodes in patients without a negative sentinel lymph node biopsy at diagnosis.[31]

Urinary Bladder

The prevalence of bladder cancer was approximately 800,000 in 2015. More than 70% of these patients were diagnosed with non–muscle-invasive bladder cancer (NMIBC). NMIBC carries an excellent prognosis but even when optimally treated has a high rate of recurrence, progression to muscle-invasive disease, or development of a second genitourinary epithelial cancer, thus necessitating long-term surveillance.[32] To guide the surveillance strategy, tumors are risk stratified into low risk, intermediate risk, and high risk of recurrence depending on various factors, including the number of tumors, size, grade, depth of invasion, and whether the tumor has recurred in the past.[33] Patients with low-risk NMIBC should undergo cystoscopy at 3 months, 1 year, and then yearly for at least 5 years. Patients with high-risk NMIBC should undergo cystoscopy and cytology every 3 months for years 1 to 2, every 6 months for years 3 to 4, and then yearly thereafter. High-risk patients should also have a CT urogram every 1 year to 2 years. The guidelines for intermediate-risk tumors depend on the specific risk factors.[33–35] For more information on the follow-up of these patients, patients who underwent cystectomy, and patients with invasive disease, the authors recommend consulting the NCCN (www.nccn.org),[34] American Urological Association (www.auanet.org),[35] and International Bladder Cancer Network[33] guidelines.

Thyroid

Thyroid cancer is becoming increasingly prevalent, at a rate faster than any other malignancy. At the end of 2015, there were more than 800,000 survivors of thyroid cancer in the Surveillance, Epidemiology, and End Results (SEER) registry. Some of this increase in prevalence may be due to over-detection of indolent tumors, but many patients nevertheless remain at risk of recurrence.[1] The overwhelming majority of thyroid cancer is differentiated thyroid cancer (DTC), which encompasses both papillary and follicular tumors.[36] DTCs tend to have favorable prognoses and often occur in young patients, so the long-term management of these patients is a particularly salient issue for PCPs. For the first year after treatment with surgery, thyroid hormone suppression, and radioactive iodine, the NCCN recommends thyroid-stimulating hormone (TSH), thyroglobulin (Tg), and anti-Tg measurement every 6 months plus periodic neck ultrasound every 6 months to 12 months. After the first 1 year to 2 years after treatment, the frequency and intensity of follow-up are guided by the a patient's estimated risk of recurrence. Many patients have no evidence of disease (NED) after treatment, and thus have a low risk of recurrence. NED is defined as (1) absence of clinical evidence of tumor, (2) absence of imaging evidence of tumor, and (3) undetectable Tg levels (during either TSH suppression or TSH stimulation) and absence of anti-Tg antibodies. Per NCCN and American Thyroid Association (ATA) guidelines, patients who underwent radioactive iodine ablation and now have NED can be followed with a yearly unstimulated Tg level and periodic neck ultrasound.[36,37]

The recommended follow-up of patients with recurrent or residual DTC, as well as anaplastic and medullary thyroid cancers, varies based on a wide range of clinical criteria. These recommendations are updated regularly and available by consulting the ATA (www.thyroid.org)[36] and NCCN guidelines.[37]

Non–Small Cell Lung Cancer

There were more than a half million people living with lung cancer in the United States in 2015, and this number is anticipated to increase as 5-year survival rates continue to improve.[1] Even after definitive therapy, lung cancer survivors remain at risk for recurrence and second primary tumors. In a cohort of approximately 1300 patients followed for an average of 25 months after treatment of early-stage lung cancer, recurrence was diagnosed in 20% and second primary tumors were diagnosed in 7% of participants.[38] Unfortunately, there are no clear and consistent data to inform the surveillance recommendations,[39] so current guidelines are based on expert opinion. For patients with NED after surgery with or without chemotherapy for stages I to II tumors, the NCCN recommends an H&P and chest CT scan every 6 months for 2 years to 3 years and then an annual H&P and low-dose noncontrast chest CT. For patients with stages I to II disease who received radiation therapy or stage III or stage IV disease, an H&P, and chest CT should occur every 3 months to 6 months for the first 3 years, every 6 months for 2 more years, and annually thereafter (with a low-dose noncontrast chest CT).[40] The American Association for Thoracic Surgery recommends continuing surveillance with annual low-dose CT until at least age 79 because patients continue to be at risk for second primary tumors.[41]

SCREENING FOR SECONDARY CANCERS

With the burden of cancer survivors increasing, there is growing interest in understanding the mechanisms that lead to secondary cancers and how this should have an impact on screening and surveillance recommendations. In general, cancer survivors should adhere to the same screening guidelines that apply to asymptomatic, average-risk, noncancer survivors, as set forth by NCCN, ACS, ASCO, or USPSTF. **Table 1** reviews the ACS guidelines for this population.[42] Secondary

Table 1
American Cancer Society cancer screening guidelines for asymptomatic, average-risk patients

Cancer Site	Population	Test
Breast	Women ages ≥45[a]	Mammography
Colorectal	Men and women ages ≥50	Annual FIT or gFOBT, flexible sigmoidoscopy ± gFOBT or FIT q5 y, CT colonography q5 y, or colonoscopy q10 y
Prostate	Men ages ≥50	Consider PSA ± DRE
Cervical	Women ages 21–29 Women ages 30–65[b]	Pap q3 y Pap q3 y, or Pap + HPV DVA q5 y
Lung	Current or former smokers ages 55–74 with ≥30 pack-year history	Low-dose helical CT

Abbreviations: FIT, fecal immunohistochemical; gFOBT, guaiac-based fecal occult blood test; HPV, human papillomavirus; Pap, Papanicolaou test.
[a] Women ages 40 to 45 should be offered screening, and women 55 and older can transition to biennial screening. Mammography should continue as long as life expectancy is greater than or equal to 10 years.
[b] Women ages greater than 65 can stop screening if greater than or equal to 3 consecutive negative Pap tests or greater than or equal to 2 consecutive negative HPV and Pap tests in the past 10 years, with the most recent test occurring in the last 5 years.
Adapted from Smith RA, Andrews KS, Brooks D, et al. Cancer screening in the United States, 2017: a review of current American Cancer Society guidelines and current issues in cancer screening. CA Cancer J Clin 2017;67(2):103; with permission.

Table 2
Cancer screening guidelines for Lynch syndrome, classic familial adenomatous polyposis, and BRCA–1 and BRCA–2

	Lynch Syndrome (Hereditary Nonpolyposis Colorectal Cancer)	Classic Familial Adenomatous Polyposis	BRCA–1	BRCA–2
Cancer sites with elevated risk	Colon (10%–82% if untreated), endometrium (15%–60%), stomach (up to 24%), ovary (up to 13%), hepatobiliary, urinary tract, small bowel, brain/CNS, sebaceous neoplasms, pancreas	Colon (nearly 100% if untreated), duodenal (4%–12%), periampullary (5%–10%), gastric, thyroid (2%–3%), CNS, small bowel, pancreatic, hepatoblastoma, intra-abdominal desmoids	Female breast (65%), male breast (1%), ovarian (40%), fallopian tube, pancreas, prostate, primary peritoneal[b]	Female breast (45%), male breast (8%), ovarian (15%), fallopian tube, pancreas (5%), prostate, primary peritoneal, stomach, gallbladder/biliary, melanoma[b]
Screening	Colonoscopy q 1–2 y starting at age 20–25 or 2–5 y prior to the earliest familial colon cancer. Annual TVUS and CA-125.[a] Consider EGD with extended duodenoscopy q 3–5 y starting at age 30–35 in selected patients, Helicobacter pylori testing, annual UA starting at age 30–35, and annual neurologic examination starting at age 20–25.	All patients should undergo proctocolectomy or colectomy. Endoscopic evaluation of the rectum (if applicable) q 6–12 mo and ileal anastomosis q 1–3 y. Upper endoscopy starting at age 20–25. Annual physical examination, including thyroid. Consider cross-sectional imaging to assess for intra-abdominal desmoids or small bowel polyps in selected patients.	Women BSE starting at age 18. Clinical breast examination q 6–12 mo, starting at age 25. Annual breast MRI starting at age 25 and annual mammogram (in addition to MRI) starting at age 30. For women that have not undergone BSO, consider TVUS and CA-125 q 6 mo starting at age 30–35. Men BSE and annual clinical breast examination starting at age 35. Prostate cancer screening starting at age 45, especially for BRCA–2 carriers. Men and women Education about cancer signs and symptoms. Consider pancreatic and melanoma screening if strong family history.	
Other considerations	Consider prophylactic hysterectomy and BSO after childbearing.	Patients with a family history should have genetic testing. Even if untested, patient should start screening at age 10–15 (see NCCN guidelines for more details).	Discuss risk-reducing mastectomy. Recommend BSO after completion of childbearing, or starting at age 35–40	

Abbreviations: BSE, breast self-examination; BSO, bilateral salphino-oophorectomy; CNS, central nervous system; EGD, esophagogastroduodenoscopy; FAP, familial adenomatous polyposis; TVUS, transvaginal ultrasound; UA, urinalysis.

[a] Endorsed by the ACS but not the NCCN.
[b] Estimates for patients under the age of 70.
Data from Refs. [44,48,49]

cancers, however, do not necessarily occur as discrete events; they reflect a complex interplay of risk factors associated with the primary cancer, including prior chemotherapy and radiation exposure, genetic predisposition, and shared etiologic factors (eg, alcohol, tobacco, and environmental exposures).[43] In other words, many cancer survivors are at higher-than-average risk for secondary cancers and, as such, should adhere to a more aggressive screening schedule. The various risk factors for secondary cancers and how these have an impact on the screening guidelines are reviewed.

There are numerous hereditary cancer syndromes that confer an increased risk of secondary tumors, either at a second site in the primary tissue affected or in a second organ. An estimated 5% to 6% of colorectal cancer and 5% to 10% of breast cancers have known germline mutations that are strongly linked with cancer formation.[44,45] Cancer survivors with histories concerning for a hereditary syndrome (eg, early age at onset, clustering of certain cancer types, or autosomal-dominant pattern of inheritance) should be referred for genetic testing, because the presence of a hereditary syndrome may affect their screening schedule. The American College of Medical Genetics and Genomics publishes specific criteria for referral to a genetic counselor.[46] The syndromes with the best-defined screening guidelines are the hereditary colorectal, breast, and ovarian cancer syndromes, among which hereditary nonpolyposis colorectal cancer and the BRCA-associated cancers are most common.[47] These guidelines are detailed in **Table 2**.[44,48,49]

Another risk factor for developing a secondary cancer is prior exposure to chemotherapy, radiation, or selective estrogen receptor modulators. Numerous studies have demonstrated a dose-response relationship between radiotherapy and subsequent breast, lung, stomach, rectal, genitourinary, thyroid, hematologic, and central nervous

Table 3
Cancer screening for patients with exposure to prior cancer therapies as children or young adults

Cancer Therapy	Recommended Screening
Radiation	Monitor for urinary symptoms and hematuria. If radiation to the chest between ages 10 and 30:[a] annual breast examination beginning at puberty until age 25, then q 6 mo; mammogram and MRI beginning 8 y after radiation or age 25, whichever comes first. Colonoscopy at least q 5 y, beginning 10 y after radiation or at age 35, whichever comes first.[b] Annual inspection and palpation of skin, soft tissues, and bone in irradiated fields. Yearly thyroid examination if the thyroid was in the irradiated field.
Chemotherapy	
Alkylating agents, anthracyclines, topoisomerase II inhibitors (eg, etoposide)	Increased risk of acute myeloid leukemia: Annual history, annual skin examination for signs of thrombocytopenia; consider annual CBC for 10 y.
Cyclophosphamide	Increased risk of bladder cancer: screen annually for urinary symptoms and hematuria.

[a] Endorsed by the ACS but not the NCCN.
[b] Estimates for patients under the age of 70.
Data from Children's oncology group long-term follow-up guidelines for survivors of childhood, adolescent, and young adult cancer. 2013; Version 4.0. Available at: http://www.survivorshipguidelines.org/pdf/LTFUGuidelines_40.pdf. Accessed February 1, 2017.

Table 4
National Comprehensive Cancer Network recommendations for cancer recurrence surveillance in asymptomatic patients after completion of definitive therapy

Cancer Site	Surveillance
Breast	Annual mammogram
Prostate	
Initial definitive therapy	DRE annually PSA q 6–12 mo for 5 y, then annually
Nodal or metastatic disease on androgen deprivation therapy	PSA q 3–6 mo Bone scan q 6–12 mo
Non–small cell lung cancer	
Stages I–II (treated with surgery and/or chemotherapy)	Chest CT q 6 mo for 2–3 y, then low-dose CT annually
Stages I–II (treated with RT), stage III, stage IV	Chest CT q 3–6 mo for 3 y, then q 6 mo for 2 y, then low-dose CT annually
Colorectal	
Stage I	Colonoscopy at 1 y; if advanced adenoma repeat in 1 y, and if none repeat in 3 y then q 5 y
Stages II–IV	Chest, abdomen, and pelvis CT q 6–12 mo for 5 y. Colonoscopy at 1 y CEA q 3–6 mo for 2 y, then q 6 mo for 5 y total For rectal cancer, proctoscopy with endoscopic ultrasound or MRI q 3–6 mo for 2 y, then q 6 mo for 5 y total
Melanoma	
Stages IA–IIA NED	Skin and node examination q 6–12 mo for 5 y, then annually
Stages IIB–IV NED	Skin and node examination q 3–6 mo for 2 y, then q 3–12 mo for 3 y, then q 12 y. Consider imaging q 3–12 mo.
Bladder	
NMIBC	Upper UT and A/P imaging at baseline, then upper UT imaging q 1–2 y in high-risk patients Cystoscopy and urine cytology as frequently as q 3 mo depending on risk
Postcystectomy	Periodic upper UT and A/P imaging; chest imaging if invasive disease. Periodic urine cytology; consider urine washings.
Post–bladder sparing (partial cystectomy or chemoradiation)	Periodic upper UT, A/P, and chest imaging Cystoscopy and urine cytology
Testicular	
Seminoma	Periodic CT A/P and chest imaging (CXR or CT) PET/CT and tumor markers for bulky stages IIB, III, and IV disease
Nonseminoma	Periodic tumor markers, CT A/P, and CXR Periodic neck ultrasound
Thyroid	TSH-stimulated radioiodine imaging in select patients TSH, Tg, anti-Tg antibody q 6–12 mo, then q 12 mo

(*continued on next page*)

Table 4 *(continued)*	
Cancer Site	**Surveillance**
Endometrial	Speculum and bimanual pelvic examination q 3–6 mo for 2 y, then q 6 examination 12 mo CA-125 if initially elevated
Kidney	Periodic imaging of the abdomen and chest Consider bone scan, pelvic imaging, head/spine imaging if clinically indicated
HNSCC	Frequent periodic head and neck examination Consider mirror and fiberoptic examination Post-treatment baseline imaging Consider periodic imaging of areas difficult to visualize on examination

Abbreviations: A/P, abdominal and pelvic; CXR, chest x-ray; UT, urinary tract.

Adapted from NCCN Clinical Practice Guidelines in Oncology (NCCN Guidelines). Available at: https://www.nccn.org/professionals/physician_gls/pdf; with permission.

system tumors.[43,47] Several chemotherapy agents are also strongly associated with secondary solid tumors (alkylating agents and cyclophosphamide) and leukemia (topoisomerase II inhibitors, anthracyclines, and platinum-based agents).[47] Screening for chemotherapy-related and radiation-related secondary cancers is currently only recommended for survivors of childhood, adolescent, and young adult cancers because the prevalence is higher in this population than among those treated as adults. Treatment-associated tumors—especially those associated with radiation—often have long latency periods, however, and can present well into adulthood.[50] **Table 3** summarizes the Children's Oncology Group's screening guidelines for these survivors.[51] Patients exposed to head and neck radiation as adults should have their TSH checked every 6 months to 12 months and periodic examinations of any irradiated areas, including the oral cavity.[52] Finally, postmenopausal patients taking a selective estrogen receptor modulator as part of their breast cancer treatment are at increased risk of endometrial cancer and should undergo a yearly gynecologic assessment.[9]

Some secondary cancers reflect the influence of modifiable risk factors like tobacco and alcohol use on multiple different organ systems, including the lungs, upper aerodigestive system, esophagus, stomach, and bladder. In the SEER registry, tobacco and alcohol–related cancer sites accounted for more than 35% of all the excess secondary cancers.[53] Among survivors of head and neck squamous cell carcinoma (HNSCC), the most common secondary cancer is lung cancer.[54] Hence, it is important that these survivors undergo lung cancer screening if they meet USPSTF or ACS criteria based on their age and smoking history. Furthermore, both lung cancer survivors and HNSCC survivors have a high incidence of second-site primary malignancies,[54,55] so strict adherence to their respective surveillance schedules (**Table 4**) is paramount.

REFERENCES

1. Miller KD, Siegel RL, Lin CC, et al. Cancer treatment and survivorship statistics, 2016. CA Cancer J Clin 2016;66(4):271–89.

2. Donin N, Filson C, Drakaki A, et al. Risk of second primary malignancies among cancer survivors in the United States, 1992 through 2008. Cancer 2016;122(19): 3075–86.

3. Potosky AL, Han PK, Rowland J, et al. Differences between primary care physicians' and oncologists' knowledge, attitudes and practices regarding the care of cancer survivors. J Gen Intern Med 2011;26(12):1403–10.
4. Hewitt M, Greenfield S, Stovall E. From cancer patient to cancer survivor: lost in transition. Washington, DC: Institute of Medicine and National Research; 2006.
5. McCabe MS, Bhatia S, Oeffinger KC, et al. American Society of Clinical Oncology statement: achieving high-quality cancer survivorship care. J Clin Oncol 2013; 31(5):631–40.
6. Survivorship. NCCN Clinical Practice Guidelines in Oncology (NCCN Guidelines). Available at: https://www.nccn.org/professionals/physician_gls/pdf/survivorship.pdf. Accessed February 8, 2017.
7. Oeffinger KC, McCabe MS. Models for delivering survivorship care. J Clin Oncol 2006;24(32):5117–24.
8. Cossetti RJ, Tyldesley SK, Speers CH, et al. Comparison of breast cancer recurrence and outcome patterns between patients treated from 1986 to 1992 and from 2004 to 2008. J Clin Oncol 2015;33(1):65–73.
9. Runowicz CD, Leach CR, Henry NL, et al. American Cancer Society/American Society of Clinical Oncology Breast Cancer Survivorship Care Guideline. CA Cancer J Clin 2016;66(1):43–73.
10. Breast cancer. NCCN Clinical Practice Guidelines in Oncology (NCCN Guidelines). Available at: https://www.nccn.org/professionals/physician_gls/pdf/breast.pdf. Accessed January 1, 2017.
11. Moschetti I, Cinquini M, Lambertini M, et al. Follow-up strategies for women treated for early breast cancer. Cochrane Database Syst Rev 2016;(5):CD001768.
12. Saslow D, Boetes C, Burke W, et al. American Cancer Society guidelines for breast screening with MRI as an adjunct to mammography. CA Cancer J Clin 2007;57(2):75–89.
13. Moyer VA, U.S. Preventive Services Task Force. Risk assessment, genetic counseling, and genetic testing for BRCA-related cancer in women: U.S. Preventive Services Task Force recommendation statement. Ann Intern Med 2014;160(4): 271–81.
14. Prostate cancer. NCCN Clinical Practice Guidelines in Oncology (NCCN Guidelines). Available at: https://www.nccn.org/professionals/physician_gls/pdf/prostate.pdf. Accessed January 10, 2017.
15. Resnick MJ, Lacchetti C, Bergman J, et al. Prostate cancer survivorship care guideline: American Society of Clinical Oncology Clinical Practice Guideline endorsement. J Clin Oncol 2015;33(9):1078–85.
16. Skolarus TA, Wolf AM, Erb NL, et al. American Cancer Society prostate cancer survivorship care guidelines. CA Cancer J Clin 2014;64(4):225–49.
17. Cookson MS, Aus G, Burnett AL, et al. Variation in the definition of biochemical recurrence in patients treated for localized prostate cancer: the American Urological Association Prostate Guidelines for Localized Prostate Cancer Update Panel report and recommendations for a standard in the reporting of surgical outcomes. J Urol 2007;177(2):540–5.
18. Roach M 3rd, Hanks G, Thames H Jr, et al. Defining biochemical failure following radiotherapy with or without hormonal therapy in men with clinically localized prostate cancer: recommendations of the RTOG-ASTRO Phoenix Consensus Conference. Int J Radiat Oncol Biol Phys 2006;65(4):965–74.
19. Caloglu M, Ciezki JP, Reddy CA, et al. PSA bounce and biochemical failure after brachytherapy for prostate cancer: a study of 820 patients with a minimum of 3 years of follow-up. Int J Radiat Oncol Biol Phys 2011;80(3):735–41.

20. Punnen S, Cooperberg MR, D'Amico AV, et al. Management of biochemical recurrence after primary treatment of prostate cancer: a systematic review of the literature. Eur Urol 2013;64(6):905–15.

21. Renfro LA, Grothey A, Xue Y, et al. ACCENT-based web calculators to predict recurrence and overall survival in stage III colon cancer. J Natl Cancer Inst 2014;106(12) [pii:dju333].

22. Pita-Fernandez S, Alhayek-Ai M, Gonzalez-Martin C, et al. Intensive follow-up strategies improve outcomes in nonmetastatic colorectal cancer patients after curative surgery: a systematic review and meta-analysis. Ann Oncol 2015; 26(4):644–56.

23. Colon cancer. NCCN Clinical Practice Guidelines in Oncology (NCCN Guidelines). Available at: https://www.nccn.org/professionals/physician_gls/pdf/colon. pdf. Accessed January 10, 2017.

24. Rectal cancer. NCCN Clinical Practice Guidelines in Oncology (NCCN Guidelines). Available at: https://www.nccn.org/professionals/physician_gls/pdf/rectal. pdf. Accessed January 10, 2017.

25. El-Shami K, Oeffinger KC, Erb NL, et al. American Cancer Society Colorectal Cancer Survivorship Care Guidelines. CA Cancer J Clin 2015;65(6):428–55.

26. Meyerhardt JA, Mangu PB, Flynn PJ, et al. Follow-up care, surveillance protocol, and secondary prevention measures for survivors of colorectal cancer: American Society of Clinical Oncology clinical practice guideline endorsement. J Clin Oncol 2013;31(35):4465–70.

27. Mrazek AA, Chao C. Surviving cutaneous melanoma: a clinical review of follow-up practices, surveillance, and management of recurrence. Surg Clin North Am 2014;94(5):989–1002, vii-viii.

28. Trotter SC, Sroa N, Winkelmann RR, et al. A global review of melanoma follow-up guidelines. J Clin Aesthet Dermatol 2013;6(9):18–26.

29. Cromwell KD, Ross MI, Xing Y, et al. Variability in melanoma post-treatment surveillance practices by country and physician specialty: a systematic review. Melanoma Res 2012;22(5):376–85.

30. Francken AB, Shaw HM, Accortt NA, et al. Detection of first relapse in cutaneous melanoma patients: implications for the formulation of evidence-based follow-up guidelines. Ann Surg Oncol 2007;14(6):1924–33.

31. Melanoma. NCCN Clinical Practice Guidelines in Oncology (NCCN Guidelines). Available at: https://www.nccn.org/professionals/physician_gls/pdf/melanoma. pdf. Accessed January 10, 2017.

32. Cambier S, Sylvester RJ, Collette L, et al. EORTC nomograms and risk groups for predicting recurrence, progression, and disease-specific and overall survival in non-muscle-invasive stage Ta-T1 urothelial bladder cancer patients treated with 1-3 years of maintenance bacillus calmette-guerin. Eur Urol 2016;69(1):60–9.

33. Kassouf W, Traboulsi SL, Schmitz-Drager B, et al. Follow-up in non-muscle-invasive bladder cancer-International Bladder Cancer Network recommendations. Urol Oncol 2016;34(10):460–8.

34. Bladder cancer. NCCN Clinical Practice Guidelines in Oncology (NCCN Guidelines). Available at: https://www.nccn.org/professionals/physician_gls/pdf/bladder.pdf. Accessed January 10, 2017.

35. Chang SS, Boorjian SA, Chou R, et al. Diagnosis and treatment of non-muscle invasive bladder cancer: AUA/SUO guideline. J Urol 2016;196(4):1021–9.

36. Haugen BR, Alexander EK, Bible KC, et al. 2015 American Thyroid Association Management Guidelines for Adult Patients with Thyroid Nodules and

Differentiated Thyroid Cancer: the American Thyroid Association Guidelines Task Force on Thyroid Nodules and Differentiated Thyroid Cancer. Thyroid 2016;26(1): 1–133.

37. Thyroid carcinoma. NCCN Clinical Practice Guidelines in Oncology (NCCN Guidelines). Available at: https://www.nccn.org/professionals/physician_gls/pdf/thyroid.pdf. Accessed January 10, 2017.

38. Lou F, Huang J, Sima CS, et al. Patterns of recurrence and second primary lung cancer in early-stage lung cancer survivors followed with routine computed tomography surveillance. J Thorac Cardiovasc Surg 2013;145(1):75–81 [discussion: 81–2].

39. Calman L, Beaver K, Hind D, et al. Survival benefits from follow-up of patients with lung cancer: a systematic review and meta-analysis. J Thorac Oncol 2011;6(12): 1993–2004.

40. Lung cancer screening. NCCN Clinical Practice Guidelines in Oncology (NCCN Guidelines). Available at: https://www.nccn.org/professionals/physician_gls/pdf/lung_screening.pdf. Accessed January 10, 2017.

41. Jaklitsch MT, Jacobson FL, Austin JH, et al. The American Association for Thoracic Surgery guidelines for lung cancer screening using low-dose computed tomography scans for lung cancer survivors and other high-risk groups. J Thorac Cardiovasc Surg 2012;144(1):33–8.

42. Smith RA, Andrews KS, Brooks D, et al. Cancer screening in the United States, 2017: a review of current American Cancer Society guidelines and current issues in cancer screening. CA Cancer J Clin 2017;67(2):100–21.

43. Travis LB, Rabkin CS, Brown LM, et al. Cancer survivorship–genetic susceptibility and second primary cancers: research strategies and recommendations. J Natl Cancer Inst 2006;98(1):15–25.

44. Stoffel EM, Mangu PB, Gruber SB, et al. Hereditary colorectal cancer syndromes: American Society of Clinical Oncology Clinical Practice Guideline endorsement of the familial risk-colorectal cancer: European Society for Medical Oncology Clinical Practice Guidelines. J Clin Oncol 2015;33(2):209–17.

45. Garber JE, Offit K. Hereditary cancer predisposition syndromes. J Clin Oncol 2005;23(2):276–92.

46. Hampel H, Bennett RL, Buchanan A, et al. A practice guideline from the American College of Medical Genetics and Genomics and the National Society of Genetic Counselors: referral indications for cancer predisposition assessment. Genet Med 2015;17(1):70–87.

47. Wood ME, Vogel V, Ng A, et al. Second malignant neoplasms: assessment and strategies for risk reduction. J Clin Oncol 2012;30(30):3734–45.

48. Genetic/familial high-risk assessment: breast and ovarian. NCCN Clinical Practice Guidelines in Oncology (NCCN Guidelines). Available at: https://www.nccn.org/professionals/physician_gls/pdf/genetics_screening.pdf. Accessed January 1, 2017.

49. Genetic/familial high-risk assessment: colorectal. NCCN Clinical Practice Guidelines in Oncology (NCCN Guidelines). Available at: https://www.nccn.org/professionals/physician_gls/pdf/genetics_colon.pdf. Accessed July 15, 2017.

50. Ng AK, Travis LB. Second primary cancers: an overview. Hematol Oncol Clin North Am 2008;22(2):271–89, vii.

51. Children's oncology group long-term follow-up guidelines for survivors of childhood, adolescent, and young adult cancer. 2013; Version 4.0. Available at: http://www.survivorshipguidelines.org/pdf/LTFUGuidelines_40.pdf. Accessed February 1, 2017.

52. Head and neck cancers. NCCN Clinical Practice Guidelines in Oncology (NCCN Guidelines). Available at: https://www.nccn.org/professionals/physician_gls/pdf/head-and-neck.pdf. Accessed January 10, 2017.

53. Curtis RE, Freedman DM, Ron E, et al. New Malignancies Among Cancer Survivors: SEER Cancer Registries, 1973-2000. Bethesda (MD): National Cancer Institute; 2006.

54. Chuang SC, Scelo G, Tonita JM, et al. Risk of second primary cancer among patients with head and neck cancers: a pooled analysis of 13 cancer registries. Int J Cancer 2008;123(10):2390–6.

55. Rice D, Kim HW, Sabichi A, et al. The risk of second primary tumors after resection of stage I nonsmall cell lung cancer. Ann Thorac Surg 2003;76(4):1001–7 [discussion: 1007–8].

Palliative Care for Cancer Survivors

Sydney M. Dy, MD, MS[a,*], Sarina R. Isenberg, PhD[b],
Nebras Abu Al Hamayel, MBBS, MPH[c]

KEYWORDS

- Palliative care • Survivorship • Communication • Advance care planning
- Pain • Fatigue • Sleep

KEY POINTS

- The palliative care approach begins with comprehensive assessment of domains of an individual's life, including the physical, psychological, social, and spiritual arenas.
- Communication and decision-making for difficult issues should include responding to emotions, planning ahead for communication needs, and considering reasons for communication challenges.
- Key palliative approaches to symptom management include addressing associated symptoms and psychosocial concerns, using nonpharmacologic approaches first or together with medications, and carefully considering side effects.
- Advance care planning includes addressing values, goals, and preferences for care with family involvement, and written or oral documentation.

INTRODUCTION

The palliative care approach focuses on quality of life, emphasizing whole-person care by addressing physical, psychosocial, family, and spiritual concerns, as well as planning for future care. Palliative care emphasizes the importance of communication about goals of care and patient preferences.[1] Many elements of this care approach

Disclosure Statement: Research reported in this publication was supported in part by the National Cancer Institute of the National Institutes of Health under Award Number R21CA197362 (NIHMS-ID: 888792). The content is solely the responsibility of the authors and does not necessarily represent the official views of the National Institutes of Health. S.R. Isenberg was supported by the Canadian Institutes of Health Research Doctoral Research Award Number 146181.
 a Primary Care for Cancer Survivors Program, Department of Medicine, Johns Hopkins University, Room 609, 624 North Broadway, Baltimore, MD 21209, USA; b Department of Health Behavior and Society, Johns Hopkins Bloomberg School of Public Health, Room 609, 624 North Broadway, Baltimore, MD 21209, USA; c Department of Health Policy and Management, Johns Hopkins Bloomberg School of Public Health, Room 609, 624 North Broadway, Baltimore, MD 21209, USA
* Corresponding author.
E-mail address: dy1@jhu.edu

(**Table 1**) are useful for internists and others working with cancer survivors throughout the cancer continuum. This approach may extend from diagnosis through to treatment and recovery, living with cancer as a chronic illness, advanced cancer, and end-of-life care. Systematic reviews support the effectiveness of palliative care for improving quality of life, patient and family satisfaction, and advance care planning for patients with cancer.[2,3]

Specialty palliative care and related services can be helpful in complicated situations, where available. However, much of palliative and survivorship care is provided by internists and other primary care practitioners, and patients appreciate the involvement of these clinicians in their care. Internists play a key role in communication about illness, symptom management, psychosocial support, and coordination of cancer and noncancer care. Many other disciplines and services may be helpful in providing palliative care to cancer survivors, including social workers, chaplains, pharmacists, rehabilitation professionals, nutritional counselors, home care, and community cancer support community programs.

Although palliative approaches and survivorship care overlap significantly, the palliative approach needs to be tailored for patients likely to be cured of their cancer. After treatment for early-stage cancer, patients' symptoms and function may improve over time, and patients may be inclined to participate in more time-consuming interventions, such as counseling or exercise. Nonpharmacologic interventions and

Table 1
National Consensus Project Clinical Practice Guidelines for Palliative Care key elements, adapted for survivorship

Key Elements	Description
Patient-family centered care	The personal needs and preferences of each patient and family is respected, and the patient and family constitutes the unit of care.
Timing of care	Ideally, survivorship care begins at the time of diagnosis and continues throughout the trajectory, including managing long-term treatment effects and recurrences, treating cancer as a chronic illness, and the end-of-life and family bereavement.
Comprehensive care	Palliative care uses a multidimensional assessment to identify and address quality-of-life issues through the prevention of or alleviation of physical, psychological, social, and spiritual distress. Palliative care requires regular assessment, diagnosis, planning, interventions, monitoring, and follow-up.
Collaboration with other disciplines	Palliative care encourages collaboration with other disciplines and services (eg, social work, nutrition, rehabilitation, support groups).
Attention to addressing patient and family needs	A key goal of palliative care is to prevent and address the burdens imposed by disease and its treatments, including pain and other symptoms.
Communication and shared decision-making	Effective communication about symptoms, treatments, goals of care and preferences, along with shared decision-making, are critical.
Delivery of palliative care	Palliative care for survivors is generally provided by internists and oncologists, but in complicated situations, palliative care specialists or teams may be helpful.

Adapted from National Consensus Project for Quality Palliative Care. Clinical practice guidelines for quality palliative care. Third Edition, 2013. http://www.nationalcoalitionhpc.org/guidelines-2013/.

tapering of medications are therefore often appropriate approaches. In survivors, medications (eg, steroids, opioids, and benzodiazepines) with significant long-term risks must be used with caution and only short-term whenever possible. The focus of support, communication, and care planning is generally different as well for survivors than for those with advanced disease, focusing on concerns about cancer recurrence or long-term progression.

In this article, we define a cancer survivor as anyone living with or having a history of cancer. The scope ranges from the effects of cancer and treatment, to fears associated with the risk of recurrence and preparation for the potential for advanced disease. As cancer survivors continue to live longer and more survivors live with cancer as a chronic illness, the role of appropriate palliative care for this group will expand and evolve. Palliative care for patients with advanced cancer, hospice, and end-of-life care is described extensively elsewhere[4] and is not addressed in detail here, although many of the same principles apply. This article addresses the following key palliative care approaches as adapted for survivorship care:

- Comprehensive assessment of the patient and communication and decision-making about challenging issues.
- An overall approach to physical symptom assessment and management. Non-pharmacologic approaches can be pursued as a first treatment step or delivered in conjunction with pharmacologic approaches. Short-term use of medications, with planned tapering when no longer needed.
- Specific approaches to 3 common physical symptoms: pain, fatigue, and sleep disturbances.
- Advance care planning when appropriate, including discussion of values and goals of patients and families. Preparation for the possibility of decision-making about advanced cancer and end-of-life care.

STRUCTURE AND PROCESSES
Comprehensive Assessment

The palliative care approach to survivors for internists begins with an assessment of biological, psychological, social, and spiritual concerns, addressing the appropriate domains and subdomains of each (**Table 2**). The domain of structure and process involves assessment of the patient's understanding of the medical situation and communication needs and coordination with other clinicians. The physical assessment includes common symptoms of pain, fatigue, sleep, and physical function, as well as other issues appropriate to the patient's specific cancer and stage of survivorship care. The psychological/psychiatric domain addresses distress, anxiety, and depression.[5] The social assessment generally includes family relationships, support, and burdens. When appropriate, spirituality and religion as well as advance care planning also should be addressed (**Box 1**).

The different domains and subdomains within the framework interact. For example, all physical symptoms must be assessed in a larger context. For pain, this includes assessments of other physical symptoms, psychosocial issues (eg, worry that pain implies risk of recurrence), social issues (eg, family support to limit painful activities), spiritual issues (eg, the meaning of pain), and cultural views about pain and its management.

Communication and Decision-making

Caring for cancer survivors often includes challenging communication tasks. Discussions of treatment options, prognosis, patient goals, and consequent shared

Table 2
Framework for palliative care in cancer survivors

Definitions	Domains	Key Subdomains
Cancer survivors are anyone living with or with a history of cancer	Structure and processes	Comprehensive assessment
		Communication, decision-making
		Coordination
	Physical	Pain
Palliative care emphasizes communication about goals of care and patient preferences and		Fatigue, physical function
		Sleep disturbances
		Nutrition, weight, body image
	Psychological and psychiatric	Adjustment
support for the best quality of life for		Distress, worry
		Anxiety, depression
patients and their families, regardless of the stage of illness or	Social	Social function, employment issues
		Family involvement, strain, burden
		Family/social support
use of other interventions	Spiritual and religious	Forgiveness, gratitude
		Meaning
		Connections to religion/religious community
	Cultural	Cultural values and preferences
	Ethical and legal	Advance care planning
		Patient preferences

Note that key subdomains are listed, but many other issues, particularly in the physical domain, may be important and need to be tailored for specific cancer types.
Adapted from National Consensus Project for Quality Palliative Care. Clinical practice guidelines for quality palliative care. Third Edition, 2013. http://www.nationalcoalitionhpc.org/guidelines-2013/.

decision-making requires frank and honest conversations. Patients with cancer often rely on their internists for direction in these areas. Physicians should use a systematic approach to communication. This includes having a plan for each time important issues are discussed with a patient, and using good skills for eliciting information and

Box 1
Palliative care principles for physicians in cancer survivorship

Care for Patients and Family Members

Provide guidance and support as patients make transitions between stages of illness (treatment, recovery, recurrences, cancer as a chronic illness)
- Provide comprehensive and competent assessments of patient and family needs
- Listen and offer caring presence
- Communicate effectively and compassionately about cancer status and its effects, prognosis, and treatment options and effects
- Engage in shared decision-making, including families when desired
- Respect patient and family beliefs, values, and goals
- Support the patient's and family's search for meaning and hope
- Provide ongoing emotional support and reassurance

Provide skilled, effective interventions that meet the patient's needs
- Refer to other disciplines and supportive services to help address needs when appropriate
- Serve as an advocate to help patients and families receive needed services
- Adjust therapies to meet the capabilities of family members, and teach patient-care techniques

Adapted from Dy SM, Grant M. UNIPAC #1: the hospice and palliative care approach to serious illness. 4th edition. Glenview (IL): American Academy of Hospice and Palliative Medicine; 2012.

communication. For example, starting with open-ended questions, such as, "What have you been told about your illness?" and, "How is treatment going for you?" is nonthreatening and allows a patient to express concerns.[6] Providing guidance to patients and families on how to approach communication and preparing questions also can improve communication.

When patients share emotions, clinicians should respond with validating statements, rather than shifting the topic or retreating into technical discussions. Clinicians should provide information simply and clearly, prefaced by statements such as, "I'm afraid I have some bad news." Good communication should address what is known, as well key possible outcomes, and acknowledge uncertainty. Clinicians should assess for understanding, with gentle repetition, as patients may not hear or understand the first time. Clinicians should tailor communication to patients' preferences for communication. Involving other specialties and disciplines can improve consistent communication and help address issues that may complicate good communication, such as family relationships and caregiver stress. Open-ended general inquiries throughout the encounter, such as "Do you have any concerns?" may encourage discussion of difficult topics and nonmedical issues, such as caregiving needs.[7]

To improve communication and decision-making processes, physicians can use history-taking skills to further clarify difficult questions or statements. For example, rather than answering the question, "What are my chances?" with an estimate of prognosis, it may be helpful to ask, "Can you explain a little more about what you are asking?" and then ask more about why they want to know. Although some patients may indeed want precise statistical estimates, others may be asking the question as a way to articulate concerns about the future or their current situation or to better plan for caregiving needs or upcoming events.

When communication and decision-making are not progressing, or there is conflict, evaluating potential underlying reasons for miscommunication can help clinicians improve the process.[8] Misunderstanding or lack of information is common, and it may be helpful to ask patients or families what they have been told by other clinicians. Key approaches to address potential misperceptions about cancer status and care include asking about the underlying reasoning or beliefs behind a decision; listening to and validating emotions; and asking about the role of the family, often a source of challenging decision-making. Clinicians also should attempt to avoid further complicating challenging decision-making by communicating ineffectively or giving conflicting information.

PHYSICAL DOMAIN

Almost half of patients with cancer, even at early stages, have at least 1 moderate to severe symptom related to cancer or its treatment, such as pain, fatigue, nausea, or vomiting.[9] Although many symptoms improve over time, some may persist. The etiology of long-term symptoms is often unclear or may be multifactorial. Patients often have multiple symptoms related to their cancer or treatment, as well as other non–cancer-related symptoms. These may intertwine with psychosocial stressors, which can contribute to the impact of physical symptoms.

In terms of treatment, little research exists for long-term symptoms in survivorship, and chronic symptoms in cancer survivors can be challenging to manage. Few large, high-quality randomized clinical trials (RCTs) exist for long-term oncology symptoms. Addressing the etiology of symptoms such as pain (eg, lymphedema) and associated issues (eg, distress) and nonpharmacologic approaches are often therefore the best initial approach. However, the time and energy level needed for interventions such as education or counseling may be challenging for some patients with cancer.

When pharmacotherapy is used, given decreased functional reserve and coexisting symptoms, survivors may be more susceptible to side effects. Key principles in pharmacotherapy for symptoms in survivors involve considerations about side effects, adverse consequences, polypharmacy, and short-term use of medications. Interactions between symptoms may make overall suffering worse, as medications used to treat one symptom may cause or exacerbate another. Issues of caregiving, spiritual or psychosocial distress, or financial worries often underlie or complicate physical complaints. Trials of interventions supported by evidence in noncancer populations (eg, peripheral neuropathy) may be warranted, with consideration of potential risks and adverse effects (**Boxes 2** and **3**).

In this article, we discuss 3 key symptoms experienced by cancer survivors: pain, fatigue, and sleep disturbances.

Pain

Cancer and its treatments cause a variety of pain syndromes, including chemotherapy-induced peripheral neuropathy, hormonal-related arthralgias, dyspareunia and myalgias, postmastectomy pain, and lymphedema related to surgery or radiation.[10] Addressing pain involves the following: comprehensive assessment of other symptoms, sources of distress, and barriers to pain management; and investigating potential related etiologies and oncologic emergencies. Although it is beyond the scope of this

---

Box 2
Palliative care approach to physical symptoms, adapted for survivorship

- Prioritize
  - What is most affecting patients' quality of life and keeping them from doing what they want to do?

- Assess
  - Thoroughly assess symptoms and commonly associated coexisting symptoms (eg, fatigue, depression, and sleep disturbance), for potential treatable causes, and consider diagnostic testing when likely benefits exceed burdens/harms
  - Is anything being caused by treatments or medications that can easily be adjusted?

- Treat
  - Discuss and respect patient preferences
  - Consider several possible options
  - If there is a procedure or treatment, what are the side effects/risks? Side effects are and risks often higher in patients with cancer, especially with chronic cancer and comorbidities
  - Balance treating a symptom with side effects and other current concerns. Is it worth it?
  - Use nonpharmacologic approaches first whenever appropriate (eg, talking about distress instead of prescribing an antidepressant)

- Keep it simple
  - Change one thing at a time if possible

- Time-limited trial
  - Try something regularly for a few days

- Support
  - Always consider psychological and social aspects, and how to work with and support the family

- Follow-up
  - Discontinue or taper treatments as soon as no longer needed

---

Box 3
Web resources for patients and families

National Comprehensive Cancer Institute
  Guidelines for patients: treatments of different cancers and supportive care, including fatigue and distress
    https://www.nccn.org/patients/guidelines/cancers.aspx

American Cancer Society
  Resources on living with cancer as a chronic illness, nutrition and activity, worry about and dealing with recurrence
    https://www.cancer.org/treatment/survivorship-during-and-after-treatment.html (Also has published specific survivorship guidelines for various cancers, which address a variety of palliative care domains)

National Cancer Institute
  Guidance on many symptoms and other sources of distress
    https://www.cancer.gov/publications/patient-education/life-after-treatment.pdf

Local cancer support organizations
  Provide many services, including support and exercise programs, often for free: search for "cancer support community" and your state or local area

---

article to address the vast array of pain syndromes, we advise that the initial approach, when possible, should include supportive modalities (eg, rehabilitation, lymphedema management) or lifestyle modifications to daily activities, as first-line treatment or in conjunction with medications. The initial approach may also include education and psychosocial interventions, as appropriate. Such interventions are supported by systematic reviews of numerous RCTs, with effect in reducing pain intensity by 1 point on a 10-point scale,[11,12] a difference equivalent to or greater than most pharmaceutical or interventional studies. A systematic review of RCTs also supports the efficacy of relaxation or other cognitive behavioral interventions and supportive counseling.[13]

Chemotherapy-induced peripheral neuropathy (CIPN), one specific pain syndrome in which medications may be effective, is a common adverse effect of many chemotherapeutic agents. Chemotherapy dose adjustment or switching to another agent may need to be considered in severe cases. CIPN tends to improve after cessation of therapy, but approximately half of patients who received chemotherapy affiliated with causing CIPN have long-term symptoms.[14] Patients may also have components of neuropathy related to other treatments, such as surgery or chronic cancer. RCTs of prophylactic agents for CIPN, including minerals, vitamins, and anticonvulsants, have shown no effect.[15] In addition, for patients whose pain did not improve sufficiently after chemotherapy, there is insufficient evidence specifically for CIPN to support nonpharmacologic approaches.[16] RCTs of tricyclic antidepressants and the anticonvulsants gabapentin and lamotrigine showed no effect, although these trials were generally small.[15] A single RCT of the antidepressant duloxetine demonstrated effectiveness, although the dropout rate due to adverse effects was high.[15] Many other agents have not been evaluated for cancer-related neuropathic pain specifically, and although the pathophysiology may be different from other types of neuropathic pain in which other agents are effective, medications with evidence for effectiveness for non–cancer-related neuropathy, such as pregabalin and gabapentin,[17] can be considered. Patients with CIPN also should be reassessed periodically, as the neuropathic symptoms often improve over time and these medications have significant side effects and can often be reduced or stopped.[15]

Although opioids have sometimes been used for cancer survivors' chronic pain, the growing literature regarding the negative impact of opioids on both patients and society warrants rethinking this approach. Guidelines for chronic pain and neurologic conditions increasingly recommend a range of nonpharmacologic approaches and no longer recommend chronic opioids, except in select refractory cases after full discussion of risks.[18,19] A 2015 systematic review on long-term opioid therapy for chronic pain across conditions for a National Institutes of Health Workshop found no evidence of long-term effectiveness and significant adverse events, including dependence (ranging from 3% to 26%), abuse (0.6% to 8%), misuse (6% to 37%), increased risk for overdose, sexual dysfunction, and motor vehicle crashes.[20] Addictive illnesses are also common in both patients and caregivers, and are often challenging to screen for and identify. Weaning off opioids started in the acute cancer and treatment phase is often an important component of survivorship care. The internist's cautious, attentive approach to opioid prescribing and management can help avoid the risks of long-term use. Evidence-based guidelines on tapering of opioids are available,[21] and similar approaches can often be used to wean benzodiazepines or sedative-hypnotics used during the acute cancer treatment phase.

Fatigue

Cancer-related fatigue (CRF) is defined by the National Comprehensive Cancer Network as a distressing, persistent, subjective sense of physical, emotional, and/or cognitive tiredness or exhaustion that is related to cancer or cancer treatment, interferes with usual functioning, and that is not proportional to recent activity. CRF significantly affects the physical, psychosocial, and economic status of patients and caregivers, as well as patients' overall quality of life.[22] Fatigue usually occurs alongside and interacts with other issues, particularly pain, distress, and decreased functional status. Symptoms generally improve after treatment, but improvement is often slow, and fatigue and associated issues frequently persist after completion of therapy.[23,24]

The approach to and treatment of fatigue are extensively described elsewhere[25] and summarized briefly here. Although fatigue is often multifactorial or is related to cancer or its treatments, the challenge to the internist is to determine whether fatigue indicates progression of underlying disease, the onset of a new medical condition, interaction with other symptoms or issues, or side effects from current treatment. It is important to identify any contribution from sleep disturbances; deconditioning, depression, anxiety, psychosocial distress, dyspnea, and uncontrolled pain or other symptoms may be factors.[26]

Meta-analyses[27] and guidelines[28,29] support a small but significant impact of aerobic exercise programs and yoga for fatigue, particularly in early-stage disease. For some patients, due to the burden of disease, treatment, or complications, exercise may be challenging or impossible. In these situations, the approach should focus on energy conservation and rest to achieve goals; rehabilitative programs can sometimes assist with maximizing function. Psychosocial interventions, including educational programs on fatigue, training in self-care and coping, and activity management, also may be effective.[30] Trials of pharmacologic agents and supplements for fatigue have not generally shown evidence of benefit for patients with cancer or survivors, particularly multiple RCTs of methylphenidate, dexamphetamine, and modafinil, and adverse effects are common, particularly anxiety and insomnia.[29,31]

Sleep Disturbances

Poor sleep can be detrimental to survivors' quality of life and affects other symptoms, and deserves careful evaluation and treatment. Insomnia is considered difficulty falling asleep or awakening during the night, which should be distinguished from general complaints about fatigue, distress, or depression. Other sleep disturbances also impact survivors, such as sleep apnea or restless legs syndrome. Insomnia often predates the cancer diagnosis, but may be related to or exacerbated by cancer or its treatments, and may persist throughout survivorship. Insomnia may be exacerbated by excessive sleeping during the day, uncontrolled symptoms (eg, pain or dyspnea), medications, caffeine, or alcohol. Psychosocial and spiritual issues and anxiety can be most bothersome in the evening and may contribute to patients being unable to sleep, and interventions such as counseling may be helpful. If patients need medications for other purposes (eg, depression, neuropathy), clinicians can consider whether medications have a side effect of drowsiness, can be taken at night, and can be effective as a dual aid for insomnia.

An evidence-based review of RCTs of interventions for sleep disturbances in patients with cancer found substantial evidence to support cognitive behavioral therapy, with some evidence for exercise and mindfulness-based stress reduction.[32] There is insufficient evidence for use of medications for sleep disturbances in patients with cancer.[32] Both the Oncology Nursing Society's Putting Evidence into Practice[32] and evidence-based noncancer practice guidelines from the American College of Physicians (strong recommendation)[33] recommend the use of cognitive behavioral therapy for insomnia as initial treatment. Cognitive behavioral therapy includes a combination of cognitive therapy, behavioral interventions (eg, daytime sleep restriction and reducing stimuli), and education on sleep hygiene, and is available through print materials, individual or group therapy, or Web-based methods. Engaging cancer survivors in therapy for sleep disturbances may be challenging, and in-person cognitive behavioral therapy for insomnia is not widely accessible, although evidence-based online programs are now available.[34]

Given the significant adverse effects of medications for insomnia (eg, amnesia, drowsiness, and rebound insomnia), they are best used as second-line therapy and for acute episodes rather than chronically. When necessary for short-term use, evidence-based clinical practice guidelines from the American Academy of Sleep Medicine and the American College of Physicians (weak recommendation) agree on use of selected nonbenzodiazepine hypnotics (zaleplon, zolpidem, and eszopiclone) and the tricyclic antidepressant doxepin.[33,35]

ETHICAL AND LEGAL DOMAIN
Advance Care Planning

Advance care planning (ACP) is the process of communication between a patient, family/health care proxy/decision-maker, and/or health care providers to clarify treatment preferences and to develop goals of future care. Improving concordance between patient preferences and the care patients receive at the end of life is crucial for patient-centered and quality care.[36] The goal of ACP is to improve the likelihood that cancer survivors receive medical care that is consistent with their values, goals, and preferences, if their illness recurs or progresses.[37] Physicians should have ACP discussions with older cancer survivors and those at significant risk of recurrence, complications, or mortality. ACP often involves completing advance directive forms to document patients' preferences about the choice of one or more surrogate decision makers (ie, the durable power of attorney), preferences for life-sustaining treatments (ie, the living will), and, ideally, more broadly, patients' other preferences, values, and goals.

Importance of advance care planning in primary care

Many patients receive more intensive treatment at the end of life than they would choose if they had the opportunity to more fully discuss their care options and preferences.[36] Research demonstrates that ACP discussions increase the likelihood that patients will receive care consistent with their preferences. For example, ACP discussions are associated with less use of intensive life-sustaining treatment and more use of hospice care.[38,39] Contrary to physicians' frequent concerns, ACP discussions are not generally associated with increased anxiety.[38] ACP discussions decrease patient stress while increasing patient satisfaction.[40–45] For health care proxies, ACP decreases anxiety, depression, and stress, while increasing satisfaction with quality of care.[38,40,46,47]

Goals of care discussions between a patient and clinician can include goals and preferences for future care, quality of life, decision-making preferences, fears or anxieties, palliative care options, do-not-resuscitate orders, and surrogate decision-making in future disease stages.[48] These discussions can be helpful to patients and for future care even if they do not lead to discussions of documentation of an advanced directive or appointment of a surrogate decision-maker.[49] Research suggests that there is a need to improve prevalence and quality of these goals for care discussions. Only a small percentage of hospitalized patients have a discussion with their physician about their future care or goals.[50] When ACP is inadequate, patients may not receive care consistent with their preferences.[36,38,51,52]

Patient-provider advance care planning and goals of care discussions

Patients' long-term relationships with primary care physicians facilitate high-quality ACP.[53] ACP is an iterative process, and professional societies recommend clinicians have multiple ACP discussions with patients over time,[1] providing adequate opportunities for patients to think about their future care through their changing health experience.[54] Patients with cancer frequently receive care from multiple clinicians across different health care settings, which challenges consistency and sharing of ACP information.[55] As primary care clinicians involved in survivorship often have a longitudinal relationship with patients and are the liaison between other involved clinicians, they are often the best to engage in ACP and goals of care discussions.

Improving prevalence and quality of advance care planning discussions

A review of communication about serious illness for the American College of Physicians found that best practices included the following: sharing prognostic information, eliciting decision-making preferences, understanding fears and goals, exploring views on trade-offs and impaired function, and wishes for family involvement.[56] A study asking patients which components of these discussions were most important generally concurred, with patients noting preferences for care in the event of life-threatening illness, values, prognosis, fears, and questions about goals of care.[50]

Successful physician interventions for improving ACP discussions include physician training, reminders for clinicians or patients, appointments targeting ACP, interactive patient education seminars, and longer times for annual visits.[57–59] However, resource and time constraints are frequent barriers to implementing or sustaining these interventions.[60] There are also initiatives to improve ACP involving nonphysician professionals and trained laypersons, such as implementing models that encourage multiple ACP conversations and communication guides.[40,61,62] Other interventions target patients through paper, Web-based,[63,64] or video tools.[65–70]

A systematic review[45] on the efficacy of ACP interventions concluded that interventions can improve the frequency of ACP discussions and documentation between patients and health care professionals. Interventions that focused on communication about end-of-life care in addition to completion of advance directives (ADs) improved concordance between preferences and the care patients received.[45]

Documenting advance care planning

AD completion rates remain low at only about a third of adults in the United States.[71] Many patients who discuss preferences for care with family or physicians have not documented their preferences, and physicians often do not document discussions in the medical record. For example, one study found that agreement between expressed preferences and medical record documentation of wishes was only 30%.[72]

States have customized ACP documentation forms and these are generally applicable across states. Several other ACP guides that have been developed for the clinical setting are also legal documents in most states. One of the most popular is the Five Wishes document, designed by Aging with Dignity, which addresses values and preferences more broadly, as well as decision-making regarding treatment at the end of life.[73] The document has been translated into multiple languages.[73] Research suggests that adolescent and young adult patients with cancer might benefit more from tailored documents[74] that incorporate language and terminology reflecting their values and beliefs.[75] Voicing My Choices is another Aging with Dignity planning guide designed for adolescent and young adult patients.[76] The guide aims to help patients communicate their end-of-life preferences to family and health professionals.[75,77–79]

In many states, when patients have preferences but do not want to complete forms, physicians can document and create a witnessed oral AD. ACP also can include appropriate discussion and completion of resuscitation orders, if consistent with patients' preferences. Examples of these include the newer POLST or MOLST forms (Physician or Medical Orders for Life-Sustaining Treatment). Ideally, these conversations and documents are shared with care teams and family members. Documentation should be placed in easily accessible areas, such as the electronic medical record and the patient's home.

SUMMARY

In summary, the palliative care framework as applied to survivorship includes comprehensive assessment of communication needs, the physical, psychological, social, cultural, and spiritual domains, and ACP when appropriate. Key principles include techniques to maximize the quality of communication and decision-making about difficult issues. Key palliative approaches to symptom management include addressing associated symptoms and psychosocial concerns, using nonpharmacologic approaches first or alongside medications, and carefully considering side effects. Clinicians should assess interactions between symptoms and other issues that affect patients, as this often affects management; symptoms should be prioritized; and clinicians should consider side-effect profiles carefully, as medications often exacerbate other symptoms. Finally, physicians should address ACP in older cancer survivors and those at significant risk of mortality, ideally through engaging in conversations about values and goals over time. When possible, physicians should document preferences for end-of-life care and surrogate decision makers, including in the medical record, and encourage discussions between patients and families.

ACKNOWLEDGEMENTS

The authors acknowledge the support of Ritu Sharma with formatting the article.

REFERENCES

1. National Consensus Project for Quality Palliative Care. Clinical Practice Guidelines for Quality Palliative Care. 3rd edition. 2015. Available at: www.nationalconsensusproject.org. Accessed February 15, 2017.
2. Singer AE, Goebel JR, Kim YS, et al. Populations and interventions for palliative and end-of-life care: a systematic review. J Palliat Med 2016;19(9):995–1008.
3. Kavalieratos D, Corbelli J, Zhang D, et al. Association between palliative care and patient and caregiver outcomes: a systematic review and meta-analysis. JAMA 2016;316(20):2104–14.
4. Dy SM, Grant M. UNIPAC #1: The hospice and palliative care approach to serious illness. 4th edition. Glenview (IL): American Academy of Hospice and Palliative Medicine; 2012.
5. Holland JC, Andersen B, Breitbart WS, et al. Distress management. J Natl Compr Canc Netw 2013;11(2):190–209.
6. Lo B, Quill T, Tulsky J. Discussing palliative care with patients. ACP-ASIM End-of-Life Care Consensus Panel. American College of Physicians-American Society of Internal Medicine. Ann Intern Med 1999;130(9):744–9.
7. Back AL, Arnold RM, Baile WF, et al. Approaching difficult communication tasks in oncology. CA Cancer J Clin 2005;55(3):164–77.
8. Goold SD, Williams B, Arnold RM. Conflicts regarding decisions to limit treatment: a differential diagnosis. JAMA 2000;283(7):909–14.
9. Silver JK, Raj VS, Fu JB, et al. Cancer rehabilitation and palliative care: critical components in the delivery of high-quality oncology services. Support Care Cancer 2015;23(12):3633–43.
10. Lynch B, Paice JA. Pain and palliative care needs of cancer survivors. J Hosp Palliat Nurs 2011;13(4):202–7.
11. Bennett MI, Bagnall AM, Jose Closs S. How effective are patient-based educational interventions in the management of cancer pain? Systematic review and meta-analysis. Pain 2009;143(3):192–9.
12. Marie N, Luckett T, Davidson PM, et al. Optimal patient education for cancer pain: a systematic review and theory-based meta-analysis. Support Care Cancer 2013; 21(12):3529–37.
13. Devine EC. Meta-analysis of the effect of psychoeducational interventions on pain in adults with cancer. Oncol Nurs Forum 2003;30(1):75–89.
14. Bao T, Basal C, Seluzicki C, et al. Long-term chemotherapy-induced peripheral neuropathy among breast cancer survivors: prevalence, risk factors, and fall risk. Breast Cancer Res Treat 2016;159(2):327–33.
15. Hershman DL, Lacchetti C, Dworkin RH, et al. Prevention and management of chemotherapy-induced peripheral neuropathy in survivors of adult cancers: American Society of Clinical Oncology clinical practice guideline. J Clin Oncol 2014;32(18):1941–67.
16. Oncology Nursing Society. Peripheral Neuropathy. 2017. Available at: https://www.ons.org/practice-resources/pep/peripheral-neuropathy. Accessed June 19, 2017.
17. Finnerup NB, Attal N, Haroutounian S, et al. Pharmacotherapy for neuropathic pain in adults: a systematic review and meta-analysis. Lancet Neurol 2015; 14(2):162–73.
18. Franklin GM, American Academy of Neurology. Opioids for chronic noncancer pain: a position paper of the American Academy of Neurology. Neurology 2014;83(14):1277–84.

19. Qaseem A, Wilt TJ, McLean RM, et al, Clinical Guidelines Committee of the American College of Physicians. Noninvasive treatments for acute, subacute, and chronic low back pain: a clinical practice guideline from the American College of Physicians. Ann Intern Med 2017;166:514–30.

20. Chou R, Turner JA, Devine EB, et al. The effectiveness and risks of long-term opioid therapy for chronic pain: a systematic review for a National Institutes of Health Pathways to Prevention Workshop. Ann Intern Med 2015;162(4):276–86.

21. Berna C, Kulich RJ, Rathmell JP. Tapering long-term opioid therapy in chronic noncancer pain: evidence and recommendations for everyday practice. Mayo Clin Proc 2015;90(6):828–42.

22. Curt GA, Breitbart W, Cella D, et al. Impact of cancer-related fatigue on the lives of patients: new findings from the Fatigue Coalition. Oncologist 2000;5(5):353–60.

23. Husson O, Mols F, van de Poll-Franse LV, et al. The course of fatigue and its correlates in colorectal cancer survivors: a prospective cohort study of the PROFILES registry. Support Care Cancer 2015;23(11):3361–71.

24. Vardy JL, Dhillon HM, Pond GR, et al. Fatigue in people with localized colorectal cancer who do and do not receive chemotherapy: a longitudinal prospective study. Ann Oncol 2016;27(9):1761–7.

25. Ebede CC, Jang Y, Escalante CP. Cancer-related fatigue in cancer survivorship. Med Clin North Am 2017;101(6):1085–97.

26. Berger AM, Mooney K, Alvarez-Perez A, et al. Cancer-related fatigue, version 2.2015. J Natl Compr Canc Netw 2015;13(8):1012–39.

27. Cramp F, Byron-Daniel J. Exercise for the management of cancer-related fatigue in adults. Cochrane Database Syst Rev 2012;(11):CD006145.

28. Bower JE, Bak K, Berger A, et al. Screening, assessment, and management of fatigue in adult survivors of cancer: an American Society of Clinical oncology clinical practice guideline adaptation. J Clin Oncol 2014;32(17):1840–50.

29. Oncology Nursing Society. Fatigue. 2017. Available at: https://www.ons.org/practice-resources/pep/fatigue. Accessed June 19, 2017.

30. Goedendorp MM, Gielissen MF, Verhagen CA, et al. Psychosocial interventions for reducing fatigue during cancer treatment in adults. Cochrane Database Syst Rev 2009;(1):CD006953.

31. Pachman DR, Barton DL, Swetz KM, et al. Troublesome symptoms in cancer survivors: fatigue, insomnia, neuropathy, and pain. J Clin Oncol 2012;30(30):3687–96.

32. Oncology Nursing Society. Sleep-Wake Disturbances. 2017. Available at: https://www.ons.org/practice-resources/pep/sleep-wake-disturbances. Accessed June 19, 2017.

33. Qaseem A, Kansagara D, Forciea MA, et al. Management of chronic insomnia disorder in adults: a clinical practice guideline from the American College of Physicians. Ann Intern Med 2016;165(2):125–33.

34. Ritterband LM, Thorndike FP, Ingersoll KS, et al. Effect of a Web-based cognitive behavior therapy for insomnia intervention with 1-year follow-up: a randomized clinical trial. JAMA Psychiatry 2017;74(1):68–75.

35. Sateia MJ, Buysse DJ, Krystal AD, et al. Clinical practice guideline for the pharmacologic treatment of chronic insomnia in adults: an American Academy of sleep medicine clinical practice guideline. J Clin Sleep Med 2017;13(2):307–49.

36. Institute of Medicine. Dying in America: improving quality and honoring individual preferences near the end of life. Washington, DC: The National Academies Press; 2014.

37. Sudore RL, Lum HD, You JJ, et al. Defining advance care planning for adults: a consensus definition from a multidisciplinary delphi panel. J Pain Symptom Manage 2017;53(5):821–32.e1.

38. Wright A, Zhang B, Ray A, et al. Associations between end-of-life discussions, patient mentalhealth, medical care near death, and caregiver bereavement adjustment. JAMA 2008;300(14):1665–73.

39. Klingler C, in der Schmitten J, Marckmann G. Does facilitated advance care planning reduce the costs of care near the end of life? Systematic review and ethical considerations. Palliat Med 2015;30(5):423–33.

40. Detering K, Hancock A, Reade M, et al. The impact of advance care planning on end of life care in elderly patients: randomised controlled trial. BMJ 2010;340: c1345.

41. Khandelwal N, Kross EK, Engelberg RA, et al. Estimating the effect of palliative care interventions and advance care planning on ICU utilization. Crit Care Med 2015;43:1102–11.

42. Azoulay E, Pochard F, Kentish-Barnes N, et al. Risk of post-traumatic stress symptoms in family members of intensive care unit patients. Am J Respir Crit Care Med 2005;171:987–94.

43. Brinkman-Stoppelenburg A, Rietjens JA, van der Heide A. The effects of advance care planning on end-of-life care: a systematic review. Palliat Med 2014;28: 1000–25.

44. Romer AL, Hammes BJ. Communication, trust, and making choices: advance care planning four years on. J Palliat Med 2004;7:335–40.

45. Houben CHM, Spruit MA, Groenen MTJ, et al. Efficacy of advance care planning: a systematic review and meta-analysis. J Am Med Dir Assoc 2014;15:477–89.

46. Tilden VP, Tolle SW, Nelson CA, et al. Family decision-making to withdraw life-sustaining treatments from hospitalized patients. Nurs Res 2001;50:105–15.

47. Lautrette A, Darmon M, Megarbane B, et al. A communication strategy and brochure for relatives of patients dying in the ICU. N Engl J Med 2007;356: 469–78.

48. Mullick A, Martin J, Sallnow L. An introduction to advance care planning in practice. BMJ 2013;347:f6064.

49. Conroy S, Fade P, Fraser A, et al, Guideline Development Group. Advance care planning: concise evidence-based guidelines. Clin Med 2009;9(1):76–9.

50. You JJ, Dodek P, Lamontagne F, et al. What really matters in end-of-life discussions? Perspectives of patients in hospital with serious illness and their families. CMAJ 2014;186:E679–87.

51. Silveira MJ, Kim SY, Langa KM. Advance directives and outcomes of surrogate decision making before death. N Engl J Med 2010;362(13):1211–8.

52. Teno JM, Gruneir A, Schwartz Z, et al. Association between advance directives and quality of end-of-life care: a national study. J Am Geriatr Soc 2007;55(2): 189–94.

53. Murray SA, Firth A, Schneider N, et al. Promoting palliative care in the community: production of the primary palliative care toolkit by the European Association of Palliative Care Taskforce in primary palliative care. Palliat Med 2015;29(2): 101–11.

54. Ditto PH, Jacobson JA, Smucker WD, et al. Context changes choices: a prospective study of the effects of hospitalization on life-sustaining treatment preferences. Med Decis Making 2006;26(4):313–22.

55. Ahluwalia SC, Tisnado DM, Walling AM, et al. Association of early patient-physician care planning discussions and end-of-life care intensity in advanced cancer. J Palliat Med 2015;18:834–41.

56. Bernacki RE, Block SD. Communication about serious illness care goals. JAMA Intern Med 2014;174:1994–2003.

57. Kirchhoff KT, Hammes BJ, Kehl KA, et al. Effect of a disease-specific advance care planning intervention on end-of-life care. J Am Geriatr Soc 2012;60:946–50.

58. Ko E, Hohman M, Lee J, et al. Feasibility and acceptability of a brief motivational stage-tailored intervention to advance care planning: a pilot study. Am J Hosp Palliat Care 2016;33(9):834–42.

59. Jain A, Corriveau S, Quinn K, et al. Video decision aids to assist with advance care planning: a systematic review and meta-analysis. BMJ Open 2015;5(6): e007491.

60. Bravo G, Dubois MF, Wagneur B. Assessing the effectiveness of interventions to promote advance directives among older adults: a systematic review and multi-level analysis. Soc Sci Med 2008;67(7):1122–32.

61. Arnett K, Sudore RL, Nowels D, et al. Advance care planning: understanding clinical routines and experiences of interprofessional team members in diverse health care settings. Am J Hosp Palliat Care 2016. [Epub ahead of print].

62. Walczak A, Butow PN, Bu S, et al. A systematic review of evidence for end-of-life communication interventions: Who do they target, how are they structured and do they work? Patient Educ Couns 2016;99(1):3–16.

63. VitalTalk. Available at: http://www.vitaltalk.org. Accessed February 24, 2017.

64. Speak Up. Available at: http://www.advancecareplanning.ca/. Accessed February 3, 2016.

65. Volandes AE, Barry MJ, Chang Y, et al. Improving decision making at the end of life with video images. Med Decis Making 2010;30:29–34.

66. Volandes AE, Brandeis GH, Davis AD, et al. A randomized controlled trial of a goals-of-care video for elderly patients admitted to skilled nursing facilities. J Palliat Med 2012;15:805–11.

67. Volandes AE, Ferguson LA, Davis AD, et al. Assessing end-of-life preferences for advanced dementia in rural patients using an educational video: a randomized controlled trial. J Palliat Med 2011;14:169–77.

68. Volandes AE, Lehmann LS, Cook EF, et al. Using video images of dementia in advance care planning. Arch Intern Med 2007;167:828–33.

69. Volandes AE, Levin TT, Slovin S, et al. Augmenting advance care planning in poor prognosis cancer with a video decision aid: a pre-post study. Cancer 2012;118: 4331–8.

70. Volandes AE, Paasche-Orlow MK, Barry MJ, et al. Video decision support tool for advance care planning in dementia: randomised controlled trial. BMJ 2009;338: b2159.

71. Morhaim DK, Pollack KM. End-of-life care issues: a personal, economic, public policy, and public health crisis. Am J Public Health 2013;103(6):e8–10.

72. Heyland DK, Barwich D, Pichora D, et al. Failure to engage hospitalized elderly patients and their families in advance care planning. JAMA Intern Med 2013; 173(9):778–87.

73. Age with dignity. Five Wishes. Available at: https://agingwithdignity.org/five-wishes. Accessed February 25, 2017.

74. Donovan K, Knight D, Quinn G. Palliative care in adolescents and young adults with cancer. Cancer Control 2015;22(4):475–9.

75. Wiener L, Ballard E, Brennan T, et al. How I wish to be remembered: the use of an advance care planning document in adolescent and young adult populations. J Palliat Med 2008;11(10):1309–13.
76. Age with Dignity. Voicing my concerns. 2016. Available at: https://agingwithdignity. org/shop/product-details/voicing-my-choices. Accessed February 25, 2017.
77. Wiener L, Zadeh S, Battles H, et al. Allowing adolescents and young adults to plan their end-of-life care. Pediatrics 2012;130(5):897–905.
78. Wiener L, Zadeh S, Wexler LH, et al. When silence is not golden: Engaging adolescents and young adults in discussions around end-of-life care choices. Pediatr Blood Cancer 2013;60(5):715–8.
79. Zadeh S, Pao M, Wiener L. Opening end-of-life discussions: how to introduce Voicing My CHOiCES, an advance care planning guide for adolescents and young adults. Palliat Support Care 2015;13(3):591–9.

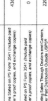

UNITED STATES POSTAL SERVICE ®

Statement of Ownership, Management, and Circulation
(All Periodicals Publications Except Requester Publications)

1. Publication Title	2. Publication Number		3. Filing Date
MEDICAL CLINICS OF NORTH AMERICA	337 – 340		9/18/2017

4. Issue Frequency	5. Number of Issues Published Annually	6. Annual Subscription Price
JAN, MAR, MAY, JUL, SEP, NOV	6	$268.00

7. Complete Mailing Address of Known Office of Publication (Not printer) (Street, city, county, state, and ZIP+4®)

ELSEVIER INC.
230 Park Avenue, Suite 800
New York, NY 10169

Contact Person: STEPHEN R. BUSHING
Telephone (Include area code): 215-239-3688

8. Complete Mailing Address of Headquarters or General Business Office of Publisher (Not printer)

ELSEVIER INC.
230 Park Avenue, Suite 800
New York, NY 10169

9. Full Names and Complete Mailing Addresses of Publisher, Editor, and Managing Editor (Do not leave blank)

Publisher (Name and complete mailing address)

ADRIANNE BRIGIDO, ELSEVIER INC.
1600 JOHN F KENNEDY BLVD. SUITE 1800
PHILADELPHIA, PA 19103-2899

Editor (Name and complete mailing address)

JESSICA MCCOOL, ELSEVIER INC.
1600 JOHN F KENNEDY BLVD. SUITE 1800
PHILADELPHIA, PA 19103-2899

Managing Editor (Name and complete mailing address)

PATRICK MANLEY, ELSEVIER INC.
1600 JOHN F KENNEDY BLVD. SUITE 1800
PHILADELPHIA, PA 19103-2899

10. Owner (Do not leave blank. If the publication is owned by a corporation, give the name and address of the corporation immediately followed by the names and addresses of all stockholders owning or holding 1 percent or more of the total amount of stock. If not owned by a corporation, give the names and addresses of the individual owners. If owned by a partnership or other unincorporated firm, give its name and address as well as those of each individual owner. If the publication is published by a nonprofit organization, give its name and address.)

Full Name	Complete Mailing Address
WHOLLY OWNED SUBSIDIARY OF REED/ELSEVIER, US HOLDINGS	1600 JOHN F KENNEDY BLVD. SUITE 1800 PHILADELPHIA, PA 19103-2899

11. Known Bondholders, Mortgagees, and Other Security Holders Owning or Holding 1 Percent or More of Total Amount of Bonds, Mortgages, or Other Securities. If none, check box. ► ☐ None

Full Name	Complete Mailing Address
N/A	

12. Tax Status (For completion by nonprofit organizations authorized to mail at nonprofit rates) (Check one)
The purpose, function, and nonprofit status of this organization and the exempt status for federal income tax purposes:
☒ Has Not Changed During Preceding 12 Months
☐ Has Changed During Preceding 12 Months (Publisher must submit explanation of change with this statement)

13. Publication Title	14. Issue Date for Circulation Data Below
MEDICAL CLINICS OF NORTH AMERICA	JULY 2017

15. Extent and Nature of Circulation		Average No. Copies Each Issue During Preceding 12 Months	No. Copies of Single Issue Published Nearest to Filing Date
a. Total Number of Copies (Net press run)		972	724
b. Paid Circulation (By Mail and Outside the Mail)	(1) Mailed Outside-County Paid Subscriptions Stated on PS Form 3541 (Include paid distribution above nominal rate, advertiser's proof copies, and exchange copies)	436	385
	(2) Mailed In-County Paid Subscriptions Stated on PS Form 3541 (Include paid distribution above nominal rate, advertiser's proof copies, and exchange copies)	0	0
	(3) Paid Distribution Outside the Mails Including Sales Through Dealers and Carriers, Street Vendors, Counter Sales, and Other Paid Distribution Outside USPS®	220	226
	(4) Paid Distribution by Other Classes of Mail Through the USPS (e.g. First-Class Mail®)	0	0
c. Total Paid Distribution (Sum of 15b (1), (2), (3), and (4))		656	611
d. Free or Nominal Rate Distribution (By Mail and Outside the Mail)	(1) Free or Nominal Rate Outside-County Copies included on PS Form 3541	112	113
	(2) Free or Nominal Rate In-County Copies Included on PS Form 3541	0	0
	(3) Free or Nominal Rate Copies Mailed at Other Classes Through the USPS (e.g. First-Class Mail)	0	0
	(4) Free or Nominal Rate Distribution Outside the Mail (Carriers or other means)	0	0
e. Total Free or Nominal Rate Distribution (Sum of 15d (1), (2), (3) and (4))		112	113
f. Total Distribution (Sum of 15c and 15e)		768	724
g. Copies not Distributed (See Instructions to Publishers #4 (page 83))		204	0
h. Total (Sum of 15f and g)		972	724
i. Percent Paid (15c divided by 15f times 100)		85.42%	84.39%

* If you are claiming electronic copies, go to line 16 on page 3. If you are not claiming electronic copies, skip to line 17 on page 3.

16. Electronic Copy Circulation	Average No. Copies Each Issue During Preceding 12 Months	No. Copies of Single Issue Published Nearest to Filing Date
a. Paid Electronic Copies ►	0	0
b. Total Paid Print Copies (Line 15c) + Paid Electronic Copies (Line 16a) ►	656	611
c. Total Print Distribution (Line 15f) + Paid Electronic Copies (Line 16a) ►	768	724
d. Percent Paid (Both Print & Electronic Copies) (16b divided by 16c × 100) ►	85.42%	84.39%

☒ I certify that 50% of all my distributed copies (electronic and print) are paid above a nominal price.

17. Publication of Statement of Ownership
☒ If the publication is a general publication, publication of this statement is required. Will be printed in the NOVEMBER 2017 issue of this publication. ☐ Publication not required.

18. Signature and Title of Editor, Publisher, Business Manager or Owner

STEPHEN R. BUSHING - INVENTORY DISTRIBUTION CONTROL MANAGER

Date: 9/18/2017

I certify that all information furnished on this form is true and complete. I understand that anyone who furnishes false or misleading information on this form or who omits material or information requested on the form may be subject to criminal sanctions (including fines and imprisonment) and/or civil sanctions (including civil penalties).

PS Form **3526**, July 2014 (Page 1 of 4 (see instructions page 4)) PSN 7530-01-000-9931 PRIVACY NOTICE: See our privacy policy on www.usps.com.

PS Form **3526**, July 2014 (Page 3 of 4) PRIVACY NOTICE: See our privacy policy on www.usps.com.

Printed and bound by CPI Group (UK) Ltd, Croydon, CR0 4YY

03/10/2024

01040397-0016